GREAT MEDICAL DISCOVERIES

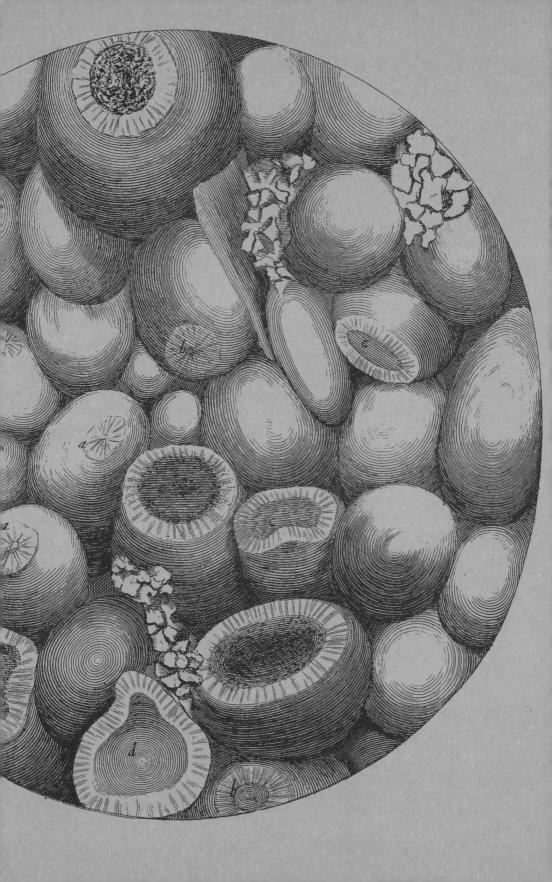

GREAT MEDICAL DISCOVERIES

An Oxford Story

Conrad Keating

First published in 2013 by the Bodleian Library
Broad Street
Oxford OX1 3BG
www.bodleianbookshop.co.uk
Reprinted in 2013

ISBN: 978 1 85124 003 6

Designed by Dot Little
Body type set in 11/15 Minion
Printed and bound by Berforts Information Press Ltd.

British Library Catalogue in Publishing Data
A CIP record of this publication is available from the British Library

Contents

'History and the knowledge of men are as much part of medicine as the latest technical devices and the knowledge of science.'

WILLIAM OSLER, Regius Professor of Medicine, Oxford (1905-19)

Introduction

Oxford has made a remarkable contribution to both the art and
the science of medicine for more than 800 years, and has had
a longer continuous connection with natural science than any
other city in England. Scientists, philosophers and physicians
periodically made the city an outstanding scientific centre of the
medieval West, and established much of the scientific attitude
and spirit that we now take for granted. Their influences and
innovations have reverberated through the centuries, providing
a continuous thread to the scientific development of today
and tomorrow. The narrative arc of this story of tenacity and
innovation is represented in the form of twenty discoveries that
have significantly contributed to the improvement of human
health. Because of the concision of the entries, I cannot claim
that they are comprehensive, nor do they represent the full
historical continuity of the development of medicine; they form
merely an episodic chronicle. Brevity necessitates selectivity,
and I have sought to choose some novel and idiosyncratic
discoveries, that merit the attention of a wider audience.

2014 is widely believed to be the 800th anniversary of Roger
Bacon's birth, and so provides an appropriate beginning to
Oxford's record as a centre of medical learning. Bacon, England's
'Doctor Mirabilis', led the way towards the conception of
science as the inductive study of nature, based on and tested
by experiment. From this foundation, it is generally conceded
that the most obvious pinnacle of achievement, before the
twentieth century, occurred in the mid-seventeenth century.
Oxford medicine witnessed an extraordinary and sudden
resurgence, a golden age of creative genius which arguably

has never been surpassed in Oxford and may well represent an unrivalled episode in the entire development of modern medicine. During the tumultuous years of the English Civil War, the experimental ingenuity of Harvey, Lower, Hooke and Willis propelled medical science into a new era. This flowering of invention was partly attributable to the breadth of intellectual perspective which informed scientific work during that period.[1] The group represented the true interdisciplinary ideal – they were the antithesis of the divided world described by C.P. Snow in 1959: society split into the titular two cultures – namely the sciences and the humanities'.[2] They were as intellectually devoted to philosophy, architecture and astronomy as they were to dissection, blood flow and brain function.

The developments of the seventeenth century laid the basis of modern medical science. As then, the last century has been punctuated by momentous episodes. In terms of human well-being, perhaps the most significant discovery in the entire history of medicine was the therapeutic discovery of penicillin in Oxford in the 1940s. This so-called 'gift to the world' transformed perceptions of medicine's possibilities and ushered in the age of antibiotics. Other diseases and causes of mortality have proved equally tractable in recent decades with rapid advances made in the field of organ transplantation and towards treatments for haemophilia B and polio. In many cases, funding can provide the vital breakthrough, as with the benefaction from the car magnate Lord Nuffield, whose many donations were crucial in establishing the modern medical school. While progress in the understanding and cure of some diseases has been impressive, other conditions remain stubbornly and tragically intractable. The immunologist Peter Medawar summed up this challenge as 'the art of the soluble', suggesting that there seems to be a certain time when scientific questions are especially ripe for answering, whereas other problems remain elusive and out of reach.[3]

One of the tasks of the historian is to remember what others forget. Medical innovation moves at a furious, impatient pace, and there may have been more medical discoveries in the last fifty years than in the previous thousand. But who today remembers Richard Lower's improved account of the mechanism of the heart or Jim Gowans's revelatory discovery of the role of the lymphocyte in immunology? These are all indispensable events in the history of medicine and deserve their place in the inexorable forward march of medical knowledge. In the modern era, Oxford ingenuity has led to life-transforming discoveries. George Brownlee's application of molecular medicine led to a treatment for haemophilia B, while the chemist Allen Hill with his colleagues developed a glucose sensor which is now used by millions of diabetics around the world. The engineer John O'Connor formed a partnership with John Goodfellow, an orthopaedic surgeon, to create the eponymous Oxford Knee, which has enabled thousands to walk without crutches. Indeed, genuine medical advances can come from non-medical origins, as reflected in Joshua Silver's invention of self-refracting eyeglasses. Silver, a former atomic physicist, has a vision to distribute one billion of his low-cost spectacles to the poor in the developing world by 2020.

The book also, in an episodic way, considers the paradigm shifts in the intellectual and scientific sweep of medicine. Oxford has played a crucial role in demarcating the ruptures and continuities in medical history. Bacon, for instance, was central to the emergence of observational science, while Hooke began work on the cell, which would be continued by Gurdon and Gowans and many others in the twentieth century. Meanwhile medicine has become ever more focused in scope, as research moves from populations to individuals, to organs, to tissues, to cells, to molecules. Basic research, clinical science and technology now work together to reduce human suffering and to increase life expectancy. Yet new challenges continue to emerge and inform the direction of research. While molecular biology has produced recombinant insulin to treat type 1 diabetes, Type 2 diabetes has increased exponentially as people over eat and under exercise. The epidemiologist Sir Richard Doll, who did much of his work in Oxford, changed the health of the nation when he proved that stopping smoking would prevent premature death. Today, as the fear of cancer recedes in the public mind, society is increasingly preoccupied by the fear of dementia, especially Alzheimer's disease.

The way forward, therefore, must be through a combination of preventive medicine and the application of basic science towards a better understanding of human biology, both in health and disease.[4] Although all medical research is by nature incremental, and its impact can take decades to come to fruition, ongoing projects at Oxford, as at other institutions around the world, point the way to future breakthroughs. Oxford's tropical medicine units operating in the southern hemisphere are at the forefront of efforts to control the spread of malaria; the meta-analysis of clinical trials at the Cochrane Collaboration gives the medical community clearer evidence of research outcomes than ever before; while pioneering new methods to discover the drugs of the future are being developed at the Structural Genomics Consortium. As the 800th anniversary of Roger Bacon's birth approaches, it is clear that the scientific methods he disseminated are flourishing – indeed, Oxford medicine may well be on the threshold of a new golden age.

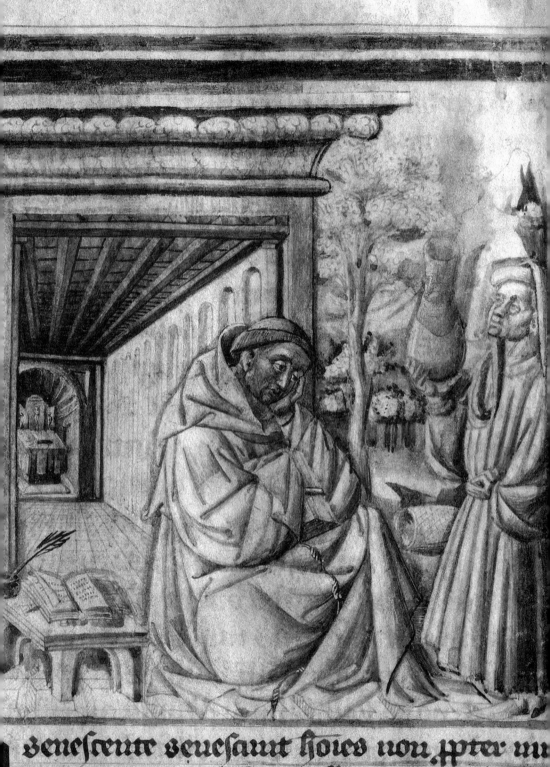

senescente senesaut homes non propter in
senectutem sed multiplicas venenau ністае
rem qui nos circumdat et uersigenia regio

Roger Bacon (1214–1292)

The origin of the scientific method

The 800th anniversary of Roger Bacon's birth provides an appropriate occasion to celebrate his reputation as Europe's first great pioneer in the field of science. Although he is renowned for his contribution to the science of optics, evidence of his standing and reputation comes refracted through a prism of obscurantism. Rather like the Swiss physician Paracelsus (1493–1541), Bacon was a noted alchemist and astrologer, and at times both men were rebuked for holding and propagating dissenting beliefs.

Bacon seems to have acquired an interest in natural philosophy and mathematics at Oxford, where lectures were given from the first decades of the thirteenth century in the 'new' logic of Aristotle. Bacon's intellect and popularity as a teacher at Oxford gained him notoriety and a position in the Faculty of Arts in Paris. Most of his early intellectual life was spent oscillating between the two cities, honing his thinking on the world of nature; much of his later life would be spent in Oxford. Before long, however, his quest for truth led to incarceration. For ten years he was kept in close confinement in Paris for political reasons, during which time he was denied all opportunity of writing; books and instruments were taken from him, 'and the most jealous care was taken, that he should have no communication with the outer world'.[5]

There is little doubting Bacon's courage for standing firm in the turbulent and contentious atmosphere of medieval political orthodoxy. An iconoclast and a

Miniature of Bacon with another figure holding up a jar, possibly of urine, for inspection, from *De retardatione accidentium senectutis…*, fifteenth century. Oxford, Bodleian Library, MS. Bodl. 211, fol. 5r.

Franciscan monk, he made a vehement onslaught against the clergy and the disputed jurisdiction between the Emperor and the Pope.[6] However, it was a command from Pope Clement IV that was the catalyst for Bacon's most celebrated contribution to science and the search for truth. He commanded Bacon to send, 'secretly and privately any writing he could prepare, notwithstanding all injunctions to the contrary of his superiors'.[7] The Pope's request stimulated Bacon into frenetic action, resulting in the completion of his *Opus majus* in 1266. Bacon brought to this work his gifts not only as a lucid observer of natural phenomena, rigorous experimenter, empirical thinker and gifted mathematician, but as a theologian and philosopher as well. For Bacon, the *Opus* was the opportunity to write an all-embracing encyclopaedia of current knowledge of the natural world, divided into seven sections: the causes of human ignorance; the relation of the sciences to theology; grammar and the power of languages; mathematics, including astronomy and astrology; optics; experimental science; and moral philosophy.

Bacon was periodically perceived as an ingenious alchemist and a skilled mechanician.[8] His contribution to the advancement of human knowledge was truly epic, including innovations in calendar reform, experiments in optics and designs for flying machines. However, it was the publication of the *Opus majus* that gave the most accurate description of his aims and labours, and made it evident that the main interest of his life had been a struggle towards reform in the existing method of philosophical or scientific thinking – a reform whose spirit and aim strikingly resembled that of his famous namesake, Francis Bacon, in the seventeenth century. Bacon embraced a forward-looking attitude and a belief in the progress of science: 'Christians should … complete the paths of the unbelieving philosophers, not only because we are of a later age and should add to their works, but so that we may also bend their labours to our own ends.'[9] Of fundamental importance to this activist philosophy was his development of the principle of experimental science in the pages of the *Opus* – he was instrumental in setting science on the path towards modernity, as an inductive study of nature, based on and tested by experiment.

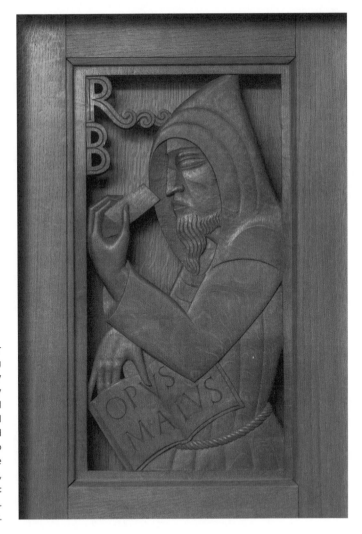

Woodcarving of Roger Bacon, depicted holding his book *Opus majus*, by the twentieth-century British sculptor Eric Gill (1882–1940). This panel is one of six produced by Gill, which form two sliding oak doors at the Radcliffe Science Library, Oxford. Photograph: photographersworkshop.com.

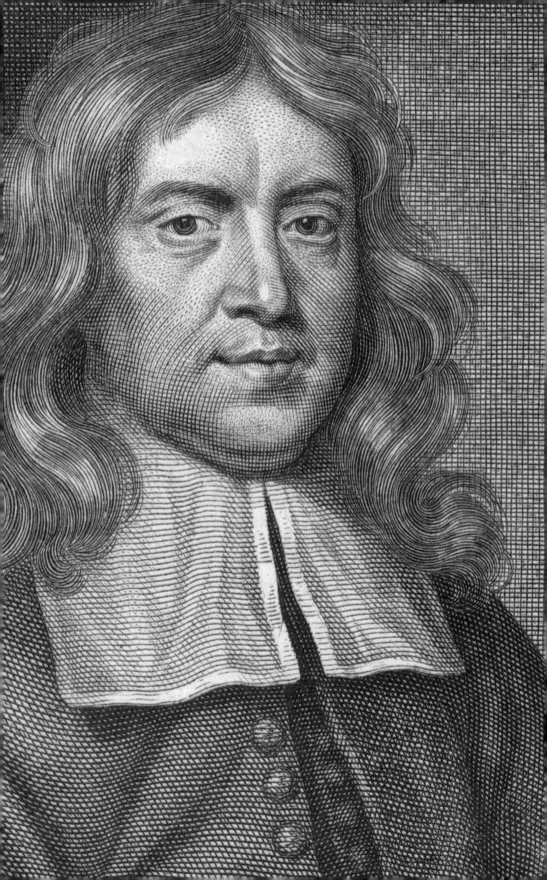

The 'English Hippocrates'

The striking achievements of Oxford medicine in the mid-seventeenth century constitutes a veritable golden age, witnessing a phase of creative genius which arguably has never been surpassed in Oxford, and indeed may well be one of the most significant episodes in the entire development of modern medicine. One hugely influential physician during this period was Thomas Sydenham. Unusually among his fellow Oxford colleagues, his reputation was not based on the experimental medicine of scientific method and anatomical dissection that gave Oxford its unrivalled status. Instead Sydenham was a champion of bedside experience. Believing that medical progress could best be achieved by discarding the trappings of preconceived hypotheses, he advocated studying instead the natural histories of the diseases which came under his care. Sydenham was acclaimed as the 'English Hippocrates', since he prized observation, avoided speculation and used his senses. Asked what were the best medical books, he replied, 'Read *Don Quixote!*'[10]

The dichotomy between theory and practice, between the bedside and the anatomy theatre, was obvious to all. Sydenham had fought in the Parliamentary forces and retained the fiery characteristics of a cavalry officer. He condemned the use of microscopes as being completely beyond God's purpose. Although this Puritanism prevented him from adopting a truly scientific approach to medicine, he was one of the outstanding physicians

Illustration of Sydenham, from *Observationes medicae circa morborum acutorum historiam et curationem*, 1676. Oxford, Bodleian Library, 8° B 47 Med., facing title page.

of his day and was lionized by many, including John Locke. Sydenham regarded the quaint combination of anatomical dissections and mediaeval disputations that comprised the contemporary Oxford medical course as valueless in training a physician for his true role of treating the sick. He voiced his contempt for the antiquated curriculum to a contemporary medical student, John Ward: 'Physick, says Sydenam, is not to bee learned by going to the Universities, but hee is for taking apprentices; and says one had as good send a man to Oxford to learn shoemaking as practising physick.'[11]

Sydenham's thinking on the practice of medicine grew out of clinical experience. Citing mistletoe growing on trees, he emphasized how disease was independent of the sufferer. Rather, diseases were specific entities which possessed unique natural histories. After careful observations of the epidemic diseases prevalent in London in the 1660s and 1670s, he ascribed their spread to changing environmental conditions or the 'epidemic constitution'.[12] He quickly became convinced that the physician should study with his own eyes, rather than through books, and that this close observation would uncover the true indications as to what remedial measures should be taken to combat disease. In 1686, Sydenham made a detailed analysis of cholera, separating it from the old descriptions of dancing mania and the supernaturalist connotations of what had been called St Vitus's Dance. He also introduced Cinchona bark as a treatment for malaria, arguably the first effective specific drug to treat any disease, while his textbook *Observationes medicae* (1676) influenced medical teaching in Britain for more than two centuries. In the longer term, Sydenham's work would later make him a founding father of the science of epidemiology, which reached its apogee in the twentieth century with the work of Richard Doll and Richard Peto.

Sydenham's observations of fever from the bedside and his treatment of the same, possibly in John Locke's hand, in English, seventeenth century. Oxford, Bodleian Library, MS. Rawl. c. 406, p. 28.

withering of ye Pustles on ye hands, wch in ye last days of this Pox (but not before) should rise up high grow big & look fresh.

De Methodo medendi morbos per accubitum Iunioris Cap 16

May ye 29th 1662 I was called in ye night to Mrs Change, whom I found very ill of a Cholera morbus, she had many ugly Symptoms, as coldness of ye Extreme parts, falling a little idly, intollerable Sickness, & felt a ting ling in her Fingers & flesh outwardly. I judge it dangerous to use Dilutients especially by Clysters in a Women soe green (she having not lain in a Month) & ye Disease pressing soe hard upon my heels; Soe I ordered her to take a warm Cordial & that a good draught of it, & her Husband to lie close to her Back naked, & her sonn of 12 years close to her Belly, & to lay on more Cloths & to warm her Leggs & flanks wth hot Cloths: She immediately fell into a moderate Breathing & all Sympt. ceased: & after enjoyning her to keep her bed ye next day, & to eat & drink nothing save a small Quantity of Barly-broth a day for 2 days she perfectly recover'd.

February 1663 I was called to Mr Halston, who after a very Chronical fever was fall'n into a very fatall like Diarrhea, I saw it was to noe purpose to give astringents seeing ye Disease proceeded from a Decay of natural heat, therefore I took this Course viz I caused her sonn a plump hot Lad of 13 years of age, & her Nurses sonn of 6 or 7 years to goe to bed to her naked, & to lie ye one close to her Belly, ye other close to her Back, wch they did, and as long as they continued wth her she had noe stools. but ye Boys rising at any time ye Looseness would immediately return. I commanded that she should persist in ye Course till her cure should be compleat (the Boys relieving one another by turns in ye daytime) & soe she fully recover'd not only of her Looseness but also of her Sickness in generall.

The very same course I took wth one Mr Little, who had a fever ab4 3 weeks & at ye time Aug: 1662 soe far spent yt his Drs judged him a Dead-man: He was ancient & having been much purged wth violent Medicaments, he was as weak as ever I saw any yt recover'd, I having to noe purpose made attempts to lay his fever by inward Medicines & to raise his strength by Cordials) told his wife that nothing could preserve his life but by putting a Boy to bed to him: soe she procured a Littl boy to lie very close to him all night, & ye next morning I found his fever almost

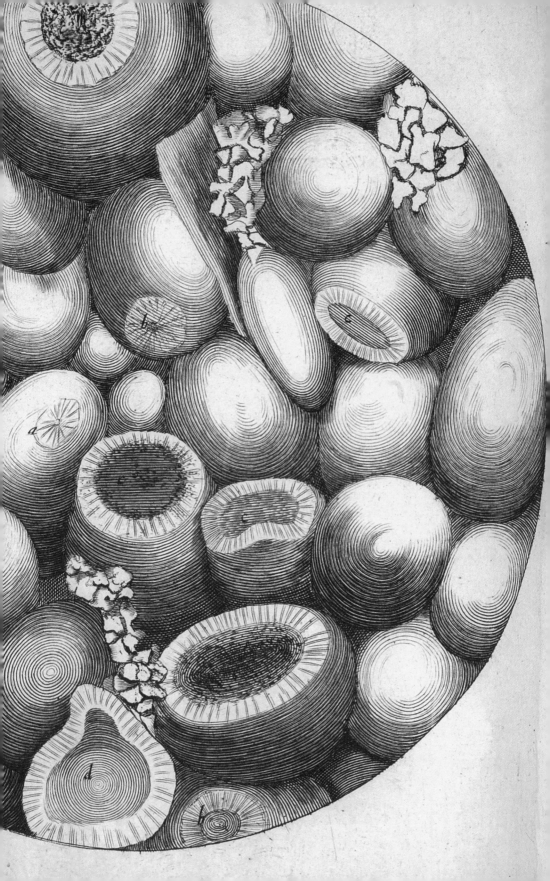

Robert Hooke (1635–1703)

Microscopy and the discovery of the cell

It is no exaggeration to claim that between 1626 and 1660 a philosophical revolution was accomplished in England. It was seen as a period of great promise, when God would allow science to become the means to bring about a new paradise on earth. Between 1648 and 1660 Oxford was Britain's chief centre of scientific activity; in the vanguard of this ferment were John Locke, Robert Boyle, Thomas Willis, Christopher Wren and the prodigious Robert Hooke. The group as a whole was characterized by youth. All members seemed to participate in collective enquiry regardless of rank or seniority: in 1655, at the height of activity during the Cromwellian period, Boyle was twenty-eight, Wren twenty-three and Hooke twenty. Hooke was the quintessential polymath, an interdisciplinary giant of his day. Medicine represented only one among many of his interests, and his great technical abilities earned him the post of Curator of Experiments at the Royal Society. But it was in Oxford that Hooke forged his reputation and found his place in the world.

The publication of Hooke's *Micrographia* in 1665 marked a watershed in scientific thought. The book was the first scientific best-seller, inspiring wide public interest in the new science of microscopy. Hooke's microscope study contained thirty-eight plates, including investigation into fleas, and featured the first biological use of the word 'cell' in describing the 'pores' of wood. Hooke demonstrated the cell structure of living tissue – but he had no idea what its physiological function was. Indeed,

Microscopy image of stone, from Hooke, *Micrographia*, 1665. Oxford, Bodleian Library, Lister E 7, schem. 9, facing p. 93.

some historians attribute this later discovery to Rudolf Virchow, a nineteenth-century scientist who worked using achromatic microscopes.[13] All earthly life is built upon, and is dependent upon, the cell. Hooke's work laid the intellectual foundations which would be built on over the coming centuries by Oxford researchers, leading to defining discoveries on the regulation of the cell cycle, the lymphocyte, somatic cell genetics, and culminating in John Gurdon's 2012 Nobel Prize in Physiology and Medicine for his work on reprogramming ordinary cells into immature stem cells.

Microscopy had become a preoccupation with the followers of Francis Bacon (1561–1626). Although the microscope was a valuable research instrument, it also provided them with considerable entertainment. Their use of it was at once a means of attracting publicity and an object of satire. Especially incisive was James Harrington's reflection that the Oxford scholars were 'good at two Things, at diminishing a Commonwealth and at Multiplying a Louse'.[14] For Hooke and his colleagues, the microscope was anything but trivial; it, like all scientific instruments, was an 'artificial organ' which could be used to strengthen man's natural organs.[15]

In addition to work with Richard Lower which verified that the air in the lungs caused the blood's colour to change, Hooke invented the compound microscope and the air pump used for experiments by Robert Boyle. Hooke's outburst of creative genius displayed during the Golden age of Oxford medicine was at least partly attributable to the breadth of intellectual perspectives informed his scientific work. He was one of the foremost exponents of the new experimental method, sometimes referred to as 'London's Leonardo' – so great was his standing as a professional scientist, architect and inventor.[16] John Aubrey, a celebrated contemporary, held Hooke's ability in high regard: 'He is certainly the greatest Mechanick this day in the world.'[17]

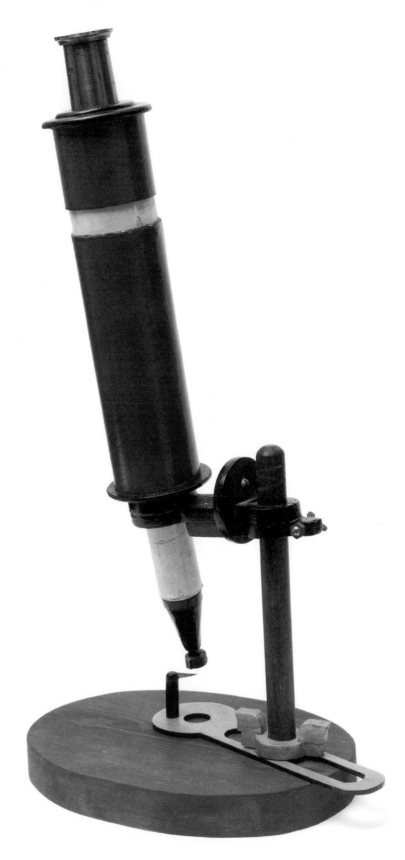

Replica of Robert Hooke's original microscope constructed out of wood and paper and containing two lenses. Made in 1975 by the historian, Professor Allan Chapman, the replica is slightly larger than Hooke's seventeenth-century microscope and is painted rather than encased by worked leather. Photograph: photographersworkshop. com.

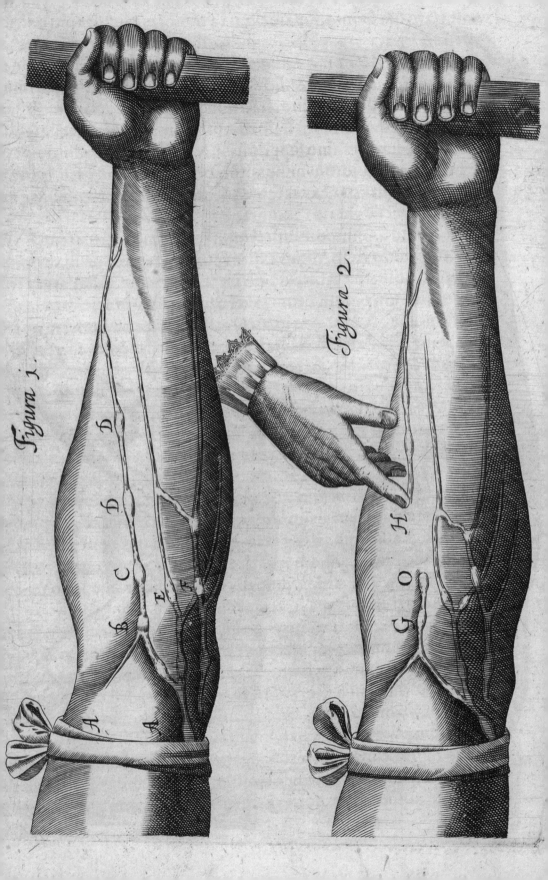

William Harvey (1578–1657)

The circulation of blood

In October 1628, a slim and rather poorly produced book was issued by an expatriate publisher in Frankfurt (even then host to an annual book fair). It contained seventy-two pages of Latin text, printed 'in tiny, blunt type on low-quality paper', punctuated by mistakes on almost every page.[18] Thus inauspiciously appeared one of the most influential books in the history of Western science, known by its shortened title, *De motu cordis* (On the Motion of the Heart). The culmination of years of research and debate, the book was the first to demonstrate accurately the circulation of the blood and the complex mechanics that powered it. Containing a dedication to King Charles I, it gave a clear account of the movement of blood around the body in a circuit. Its impact, and that of its author William Harvey, was, according to Harvey's latest biographer, 'arguably as great as Darwin's theory of evolution and Newton's theory of gravity'.[19]

Harvey's name is rightly at the forefront of medical history, for he applied experimental methods to discover the circulation of blood. Together with continental counterparts including Descartes, Galileo, Kepler and Mersenne, he unleashed a tidal wave of experimental science across Europe. In 1600, he travelled to Padua, joining a long list of sixteenth-century English alumni which included Thomas Wyatt, Sir Philip Sidney and Sir Francis Walsingham. There he studied under Girolamo Fabreizie da Acquaponte (or Fabricius), and watched

Blood flow in the forearm, from Harvey, *De motu cordis*, 1628. Oxford, Bodleian Library, 4° H 3 Med. Seld., plate 1 after p. 56.

him dissect dead criminals and living animals in the university's famous Teatro Anatomico. Harvey's own pre-eminence in public dissections was much talked of. He was 'unrivalled at the table', wrote one spectator; he had 'dexterity beyond compare'.[20] Key to the success of Harvey's later work was the formative period of education in Italy, where he turned to nature as the source of material scientific truth. 'I do not profess', he was to write later, 'to learn and teach anatomy from the axioms of philosophies but from dissections, and from the fabrick of Nature.'[21]

Anatomical studies, particularly the dissection of corpses for teaching and research, were commonplace in Europe's universities, yet the fundamental understanding of the workings of physiology had changed little for centuries. The doggedly orthodox College of Physicians still championed the classical precepts of Galen, and Harvey proceeded cautiously in his disproval of them. When his dissections pointed to the inadequacy of Galenic theories of the heart and blood, he tactfully suggested that the human body had changed since Roman times. Harvey's key interest lay in the area of hydraulics. Tradition taught that arteries had an active pulsatory force, but Harvey realized they were passive, like the lead pipes of London's rapidly developing water system. Arterial blood was solely pumped around the body by the heart's 'vigourous beat' – and this perception of the heart as a piece of robust but intricate machinery was to have a profound influence on the new generation of Neoteric or mechanistic philosophers such as Descartes.[22]

Harvey spent only four years in Oxford, but for him, as for so many of his contemporaries, they were momentous years. Harvey arrived in Oxford as physician to the King, and his fame went some way to reinvigorating the medical faculties and their students.

Prescription by Harvey for John Aubrey, for a 'purge to prevent an impostumation [abscess]'. Oxford, Bodleian Library, MS. Aubrey 21, fol. 112.

The list of alumni who either assisted Harvey or went on to make significant contributions to research on circulation, applying Harvey's techniques in the wider fields of anatomy and physiology, is striking. These students and many other enthusiasts for experimental physiology came into direct contact with Harvey when he served as Warden of Merton College between 1642 and 1646. This period was spent consolidating work on *De generatione*, Harvey's great treatise on embryology, which was published in 1651.

ruofum finum vi injiciatur, mox enim confpicietur, prope glandulam pitui-tariam diverfis in locis erumpere at-que fcaturire: certo utique indicio, quicquid feri a cerebro fecernitur, in fanguinem denuò refundi, eique com-mifceri.

CAP. III.

Sanguinis Motus & Color.

De celeritate circulationis & quæ fit differentia inter fanguinem venofum & arteriofum.

Poftquam ad hunc modum con-ftitit qualis cordis fabrica fit, unde ejus motus provenit, qui-bufque de caufis motus ejus alteretur, & quales effectus & fymptomata alte-rationes iftæ fanguini inducant, reftat ut quàm celeri curfu fanguis omnis per cor circuletur proximè oftendam.

De

De motu fanguinis per ventriculos cordis quæcunque ante *Harveium* au-thores tradiderunt, tam inania & futilia funt ut fponte fuâ jam evanuerint: Quinimò & inter pofteros qui in-ventam ab ipfo circulationem amplexi funt, utcunque, ipfa hypothefi cogen-te, totum fanguinem tranfire cor & circulari ftatuunt, de tranfitûs tamen celeritate & quantitate fanguinis qua-libet vibratione expreffi ita fcripferunt, ut fabricam cordis motufque ejus non fatis attendiffe videantur: Nam ple-rique guttulas aliquot, aut fcrupulum, aut drachmam unam, pauci femiün-ciam tantùm fanguinis fingulis pulfi-bus expelli concedunt. Et quidem fatendum eft in diverfis animalibus pro variâ corporis magnitudine, cordis ventriculos plus aut minus continere & ejicere; verum in homine aut ma-jore quovis animali tam exiguam quan-titatem quolibet pulfu tranfmitti, quàm fit inconfultum afferere ex fequentibus patebit.

Equidem in eâ opinione fum totam fanguinis maffam qualibet horâ non felem

Richard Lower (1631–1691)

Blood, transfusions
and respiration

Richard Lower was a distinguished member of the
scientific community which flourished in Oxford
from 1643 to 1667, many of whose members later
migrated to London to form the nucleus of the Royal
Society. Lower made notable contributions in the
study of anatomy and physiology and also practised
medicine, eventually becoming the leading London
physician of his day. He was an expert anatomist, a fact
acknowledged by Thomas Willis, Sedleian Professor
of Natural Philosophy 'when we were entering upon a
much more difficult task, the dissection of the nerves,
the really wonderful dexterity of this worker and his
untiring perseverance were conspicuous in the extreme
and no obstacle could withstand his effort…'[23] In spite
of his achievements, however, Lower remains largely
unknown, being overshadowed by his illustrious
contemporaries, who included Willis, Robert Boyle,
John Locke and Robert Hooke.

The revolutionary decades 1640–60 had profound
effects on the course of English physiology. For a brief
period, the writings of Oxford physiologists suddenly
projected Britain to the zenith of international medical
research. Key to Oxford's contribution to seventeenth-
century medicine was the work of Lower, whose detailed
account of the mechanism of the heart built upon
William Harvey's earlier work, and was published as
Tractatus de corde in 1669. Harvey's discovery of the
circulation of the blood combined with the experimental

'Sanguinis Motus &
Color', discussing the
oxygenation of the blood,
Lower, *Tractatus de corde*,
1669. Oxford, Bodleian
Library, 8° V 15 Med., pp.
152-3.

nature of the Oxford natural philosophers provided a new impetus for an attempt at transfusion of blood from one animal to another. In 1667, Lower, in collaboration with Edmund King, performed the first human blood transfusion in England, just five months after Jean Denis had performed the first such operation on a human in Paris. Lower managed to persuade former Cambridge student Arthur Coga to undergo a transfusion of sheep's blood. Surprisingly, Coga survived the procedure and less than a month later the demonstration was repeated for the benefit of the Fellows of the Royal Society, with Coga himself describing the effects of the transfusion.

The function of respiration and its relationship to the change in colour between arterial and venous blood had stimulated the research efforts of Lower and others. In October 1667, Lower and Robert Hooke conducted an experiment showing that on opening the pulmonary

Medical notebook of John Locke containing prescriptions attributed to Richard Lower, but in Locke's hand, written in English. Oxford, Bodleian Library, MS. Locke e. 4, pp. 24-25.

vein, florid red blood emerged, indicating that the blood's colour change took place in the lungs, and not in the left ventricle as previous believed. If the animal (in this case a dog) was asphyxiated, the pulmonary vein blood remained purple, showing that whatever entered the blood in the pulmonary transit to effect the colour change was essential to life. Thus Lower was the first man in medical history to explain the cause of the change in colour of the blood. In 1669, Lower published *Tractatus de corde*, a summary of his finest anatomical and physiological achievements, which is rightly regarded as a medical classic. However, it was a considerable time before the full implications of Lower's accomplishments, most notably the transfusion of blood and the explanation for the differing colour of arterial blood, were realized. Lower was certainly a man of his time but his insights, formed by experimentation, still resonate down the centuries.

Anser: et Anat ana Ʒiſs. diſſolvantur permiſcendo.
senſim olibani ℔ſs postquam fervore desierint adde
pulvriſ Cumini Ʒij piper Ʒſs ol. Spic. Ʒſ fiat
emplaſtrum ot plantiſ ni socciſ lineiſ applicetur. adhareat
2ª Sephimanaſ Plateruſ
Si dolor fiat acrior difeendentiſ humoriſ niunge Krura
obro nervino hypouti mr Lower.

✝ Dysentria vd Besborum.

Chiromant. La Chambre. Chiromantia
The Bart will not grow soft ni bai Brig un lſſr : the
carſ br cut off
The fore fringor Rat a sympathy wt yr livor yr 2d wt yr
gelovne yr 3d wt yr Bart
The Leprosy Rat its fourſt e prmciplr wal ni yr Livor et
firel signr wbrcbſ li hounr apparſ ni yr fore fringor for

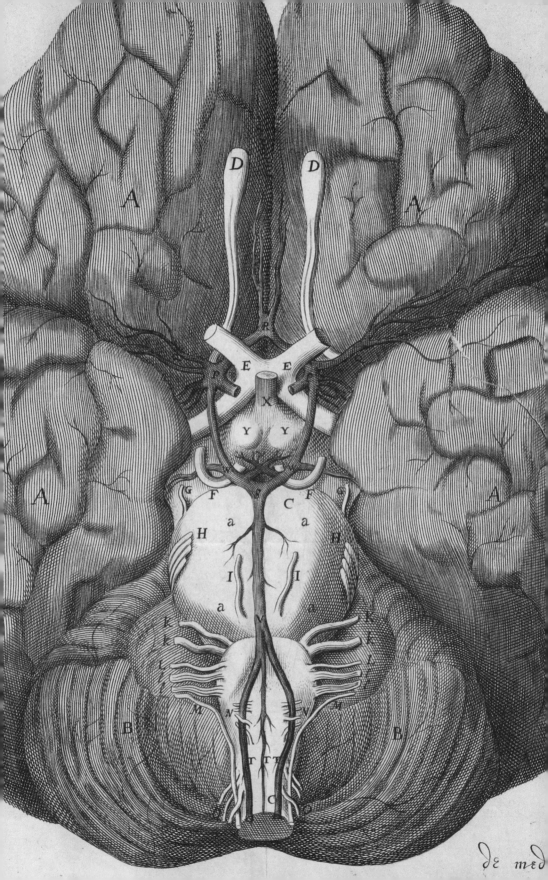

de med

The beginnings of neurology

Thomas Willis (1621–1675)

The seizure of Oxford by Cromwell's Parliamentary forces in 1646 prompted a Royalist exodus. The King's supporters either left Oxford voluntarily or were forcibly expelled. Despite this, one of the leading researchers of the seventeenth century, Thomas Willis, confounded the trend by forging a successful career in the new Parliamentarian stronghold. Although a staunch Royalist, Willis remained in Oxford as a practising doctor, which included a regular practice in Abingdon market, before he was appointed Sedleian Professor at the University during the Restoration in 1660.

Along with Hooke and Lower, Willis remains a giant in the field of early modern scientific research. His writings on the brain and the nervous system were key discoveries in the advancement of fledgling medical knowledge and practice, and occupy a prominent position in the legacy of Oxford medicine in the seventeenth century. Like Sydenham, Willis was fortunate in his formal medical training. It was brief. He avoided the dull, classical medical texts, and, as an early member of an experimental philosophical club – which later became the Royal Society – immersed himself instead in dissections, experiments and discussions. Self-taught, Willis coined the word 'neurologie', which first appeared in his book *Cerebri anatome* in 1664, and in English in 1681. The genesis of the book came from Willis's decision to undertake a new study of the anatomy of the brain in order to understand the functions of the

Diagram by Christopher Wren, illustrating the Circle of Willis, from Willis, *Cerebri anatome*, 1664. Oxford, Bodleian Library, 4° Q 7 Med., figure 1.

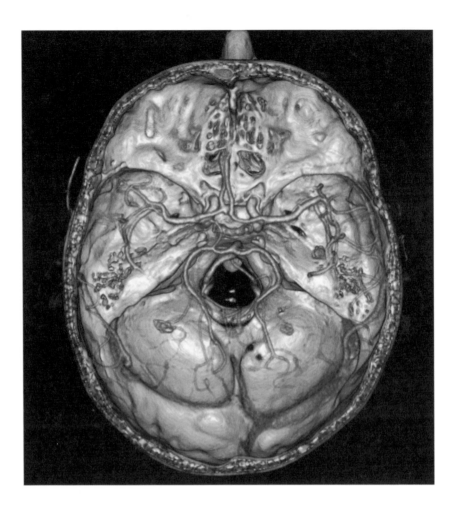

cerebellum and the pathogenesis of dysfunctions such as
paralysis, insomnia, epilepsy, hysteria and convulsions.
In 1661, Willis began his project on the cerebral
circulation by injecting a liquid dye 'with saffron, and
other colours into the arterial carotides' so as 'to try how
the blood moves'.[24] Meanwhile, in the Auctorium of the
Bodleian Library (then part of the School of Medicine)
human cadavers, horses, dogs, cats, fish and sheep were
dissected with the help of Christopher Wren and Richard
Lower. Wren would also provide the series of illustrations
of the arterial circle at the base of the brain which helped

Contemporary
image of the Circle of
Willis, produced by
the Department of
Neuroradiology, John
Radcliffe Hospital,
Oxford. Image courtesy
of James V. Byrne FRCS
FRCR, Professor of
Neuroradiology.

to make *Cerebri anatome* the most advanced text of neuroanatomy of the age.

Cerebri anatome is chiefly remembered for this first complete description of the arterial circle at the base of the brain, the 'circle of Willis', although this eponymous label was attached later by the Swiss anatomist, Albrecht von Haller. Willis's delineation of the peripheral and autonomic nervous system was matched only by his pioneering work on the brain and spinal cord: he was the first to describe and illustrate the brain from accurate observation, and his descriptive terms – for example cerebral peduncles and medullary pyramids – persist to this day.

Willis died in 1675, at the age of fifty-four. His lasting memorial is to be found in the work of Nathaniel Williams, in an elegy published in 1675. After reviewing his writings on fevers, chemistry and therapeutics, the poet acclaims Thomas Willis's *Cerebri anatome* in verse:

> *Thou knewst the wondrous art,*
> *And order of each part*
> *In the whole lump, how every sense*
> *Contributes to the healths defence.*
> *The several channels, which convey*
> *The vital current every way;*
> *Trackst wise nature everywhere,*
> *In every region, every sphere,*
> *Fathomst the mistery,*
> *Of deep Anatomy;*
> *Thunactive carcas thou hast preyd upon,*
> *And stript it to a sceleton,*
> *But now (alas!) the art is gone,*
> *And now on thee,*
> *The crawling worms experience their Anatomy.*[25]

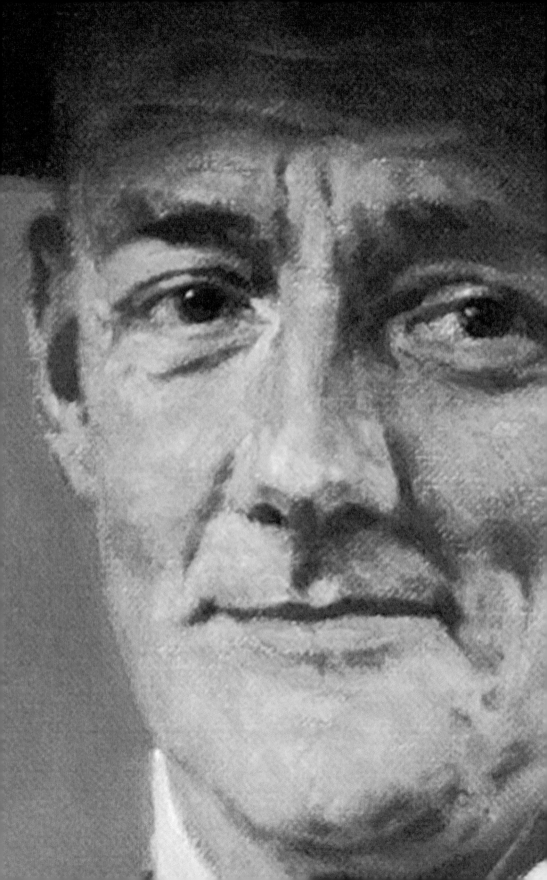

The Nuffield Benefaction

Laying the foundations of the Oxford Medical School

Oxford, unlike Cambridge, had an industrial revolution in the twentieth century. William Morris (1877–1963), later known as Lord Nuffield, transformed Oxford into one of the world's leading centres of car manufacturing.[26] By the middle decades of the twentieth century, more than 28,000 people worked at the Cowley car factory, while Nuffield's eponymous sports cars, MG (Morris Garages), were lionized throughout Europe and North America. By the middle of the 1930s, Nuffield was one of the nation's richest industrialists. Like his American contemporaries Rockefeller and Carnegie, he used his accumulated capital for philanthropic purposes. He embraced Winston Churchill's aphorism, 'We make a living by what we get, but we make a life by what we give.'[27]

Nuffield was a lifelong hypochondriac. This anxiety about his health stimulated an early interest in medicine and led him to make friendships within the medical profession, first with William Osler, the Regius Professor of Medicine at Oxford (1905–1919) and later with Farquhar Buzzard, (Regius Professor 1928–43), Gathorne Girdlestone, orthopaedic surgeon, Robert Macintosh, anaesthetist and Hugh Cairns, neurosurgeon." In 1936 Nuffield wrote to the Vice Chancellor of Oxford University that 'the progress of medical science and the conditions under which medical practice is carried on have long been among my main interests.'[28] He donated £2 million – a benefaction on an industrial scale, equivalent to over £1 billion today. Nuffield's generosity

Portrait of Lord Nuffield, currently displayed at the John Radcliffe Hospital, Oxford. Photograph: photographersworkshop. com.

had a dramatic effect on Oxford medicine, laying the modern foundations of the Oxford Medical School. His first donation to Oxford medicine was used to found the Nuffield Institute for Medical Research, located in the old Oxford Observatory. The development of the Observatory as a research institute was intimately linked to the development of the Medical School. Hugh Cairns, having spent a year with Harvey Cushing at Harvard, became taken with the idea of creating a school of medicine at Oxford.[29] Nuffield's money was very well spent. By the end of the 1930s, five new chairs had been established and the outstanding quality of the appointments heralded a new era in clinical care in Oxford. The development of the school of medicine included five Nuffield professors: clinical medicine (Witts), obstetrics and gynaecology (Chassar Moir), surgery (Cairns), orthopaedics (Girdlestone) and anaesthetics. The last position was particularly visionary, as its occupant, Macintosh, was the first Professor of Anaesthetics in Europe.

Nuffield was a contradictory and controversial figure. He had an antipathy for the trade-union movement and the status of industrial relations at his factories was often neuralgic. Moreover, his support for Oswald Mosley's British Union of Fascists did not serve him well and reflected a naivety and contempt that were at odds with the national mood.

On the other hand, he was deeply moved by the Hippocratic ideal of healing the sick and to this cause he was untiringly devoted. From an early age, he had wanted to be a doctor. While this failure was a source of lingering personal disappointment, it was to Oxford medicine's great good fortune.

The Observatory building at Green Templeton College, Oxford. Medical scientists within the Nuffield Institute of Medical Research moved into the building in 1934, following its purchase in 1930 by Sir William Morris (later Lord Nuffield), who presented it to the University. Image courtesy of Green Templeton College, Oxford.

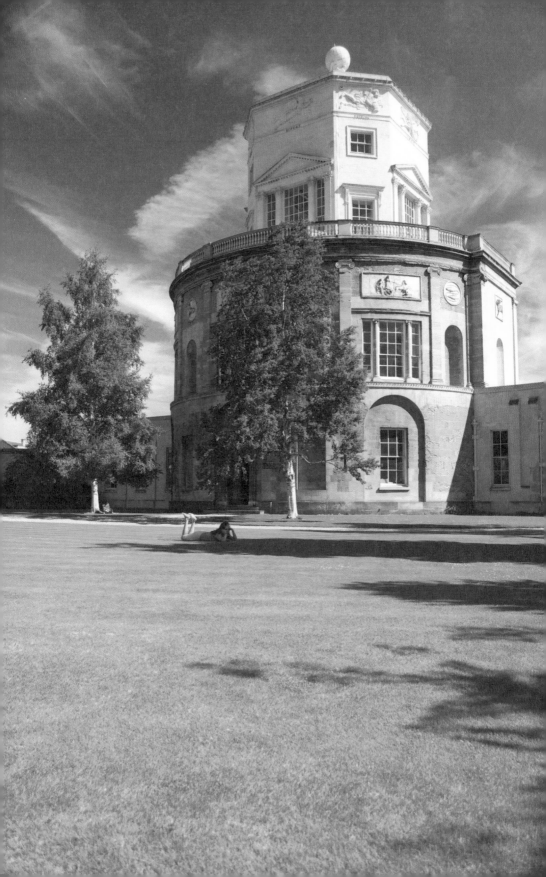

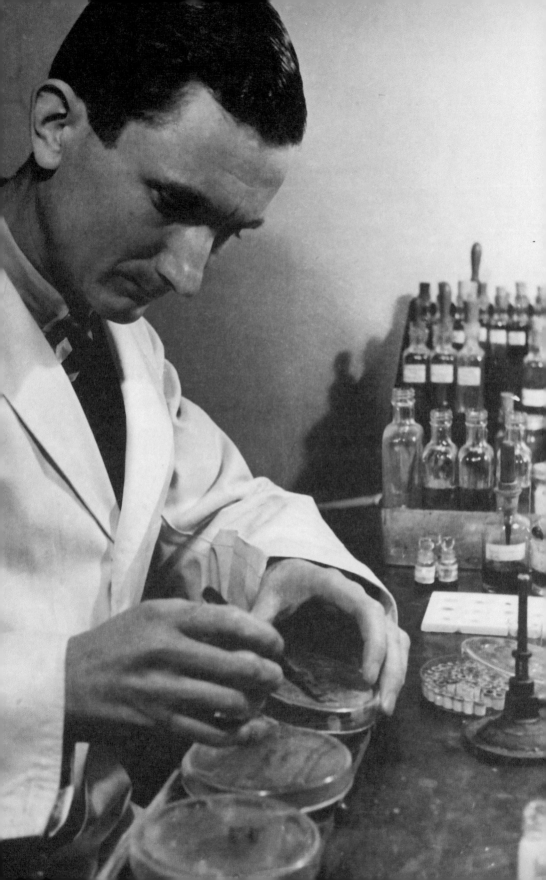

Penicillin

A gift to the world

The development of penicillin is one of the greatest stories in biomedical history. More than any other drug, penicillin liberated the art of medicine from its ineffectiveness against disease and brought a cure for the lethal common infections of pneumonia, meningitis and septicaemia. This breakthrough may be regarded as the true dawn of the age of antibiotics, which have since transformed doctors' and society's perceptions of medicine's possibilities.

Alexander Fleming's discovery of penicillin is well known. Less familiar is the crucial and inspiring work of scientists at Oxford University which, in the 1940s, led to penicillin being transformed into a therapeutic drug that would save millions of lives. The limited resources of wartime Britain taxed scientists' skills and inventiveness to the full, and meant that British firms could not undertake commercial production. But from an ingeniously improvised production line, the Oxford team succeeded in producing enough of the drug to demonstrate its miraculous potential. The team then shared its knowledge with American pharmaceuticals companies, enabling the mass production of penicillin in time for the last stages of World War II. In honour of their work, Alexander Fleming and two members of the Oxford team, Howard Florey and Ernst Chain, shared the 1945 Nobel Prize in Physiology or Medicine 'for the discovery of penicillin and its curative effects in various infectious diseases'.

The biochemist Norman Heatley (1911–2004) working in the Sir William Dunn School of Pathology, Oxford. By early 1941, large areas of the Dunn School had been turned into a factory with mechanical apparatus designed by Heatley for extracting the penicillin. Image courtesy of the Sir William Dunn School of Pathology, Oxford.

The decisive work took place under Florey, Chain, Norman Heatley and others at the Sir William Dunn School of Pathology. While Heatley was not awarded a Nobel Prize, his work is rightly regarded as pivotal in the penicillin story.[30] Heatley was a biochemist with the hands of a neurosurgeon, a master of invention, who with dexterous skills and practical mind constructed futuristic apparatus that produced the elusive antibiotic which revolutionized biomedical science. Florey, the Australian team leader, was uncompromising, dedicated and single-minded. According to Jim Gowans, one of Florey's DPhil students, Florey didn't like speculation – 'the thing he liked most was the simple, telling experiment'.[31] This was exactly what Heatley was able to provide on 25 May 1940. Eight mice were given a lethal dose of the streptococci bacteria – four of the eight were then given penicillin. The protective effects of the drug result were stunning. When Florey, returning to the lab with Chain after a dinner together at Lincoln College, saw the preliminary result, he described it as a miracle.[32] So great was Heatley's humanity that he took the four dead mice to his home, wrapped them in some of his children's unwanted clothes, and buried them in his flower garden.[33]

Such was the value of Heatley's contribution that in 1990, he was awarded the unusual distinction of an honorary doctorate of medicine from Oxford University, the first given to a non-medic in Oxford's 800-year history. During the ceremony, the lean, seventy-nine-year-old biochemist was described as 'a virtual Hercules'.[34] Assessing the contributions of the main protagonists in the penicillin story, Professor Sir Henry Harris, former head of the Sir William Dunn School of Pathology, stated in 1998: 'Without Fleming, no Chain or Florey; without Chain, no Florey; without Florey, no Heatley; without Heatley, no penicillin.'[35]

Photograph of penicillin sodium salt crystal. Oxford, Bodleian Library, MS. Eng. c 5604/17

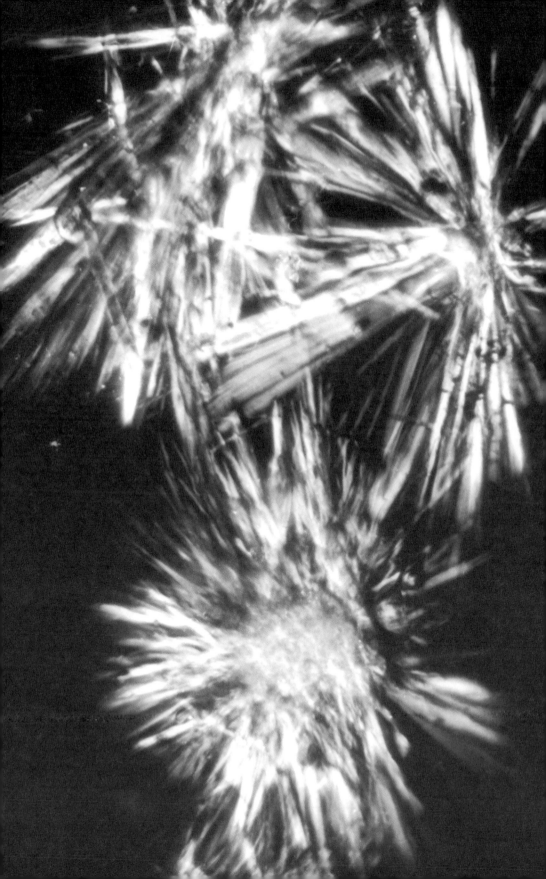

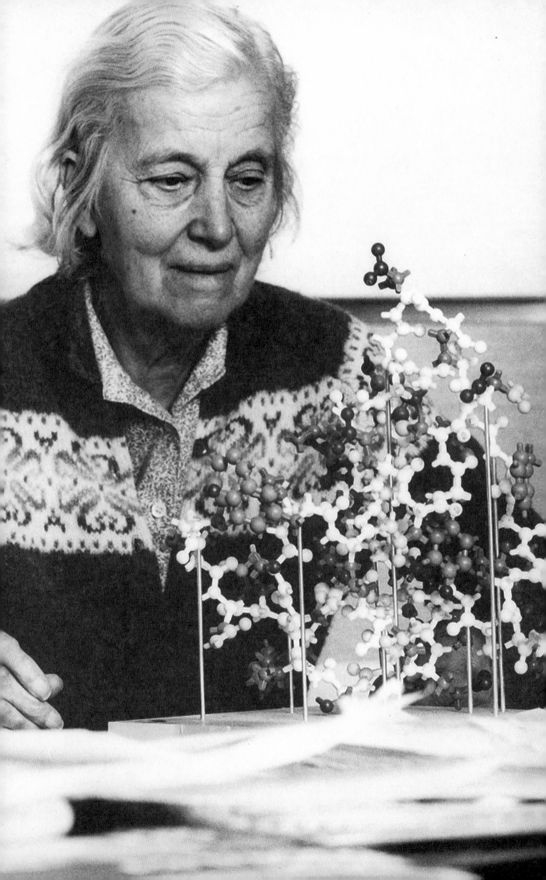

Dorothy Hodgkin

Britain's only female Nobel Prize winner in science

Dorothy Hodgkin was one of the most remarkable and successful chemists of the twentieth century, discovering the structures of penicillin, insulin and vitamin B12 through her pioneering use of crystallography. As a young girl, Dorothy first encountered chemistry, growing crystals of alum and copper sulphate. She later recalled, 'I was captured for life by chemistry and by crystals.'[36] Hodgkin (née Crowfoot) read for a degree in chemistry at Somerville College, Oxford, in 1928. In 1932, she moved to the University of Cambridge and did doctoral work under the supervision of the visionary physicist John Desmond Bernal. In Bernal's laboratory, she helped him to make the first X-ray diffraction studies of pepsin, a crystalline protein. She returned to Oxford and to Somerville in 1934, where she remained until retirement in 1974. Her prodigious output not only supercharged Oxford science in general, but also signposted the way forward for chemists, crystallographers and biologists.

In 1941, when Howard Florey and his team at the William Dunn School succeeded in isolating penicillin, they asked Hodgkin to 'solve', or map, its molecular structure. By 1945, she had accomplished the task, describing the arrangement of its atoms in three dimensions. The importance of her work was recognized by election to the Royal Society in 1947, only two years after the first woman had been elected. Science at Oxford was very much a male preserve, but Hodgkin's pioneering brilliance shone through – not only did her own career flourish, but she also became

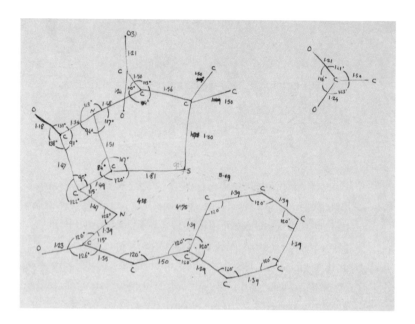

an inspirational figure to other women seeking a life in experimental science. Famously, Margaret Roberts enrolled at Somerville as a chemistry student to learn directly from Hodgkin, and later, as Margaret Thatcher, became the first woman and first scientist to be elected prime minister.

Hodgkin established her own laboratory in a cramped, crypt-like room in a corner of the Oxford University Museum of Natural History and it was from here that she forged her reputation as a founder of the science of protein crystallography. The challenges were colossal, as every new technique seemed to reach limits that constrained the size of the protein that could be successfully solved, and each protein tackled presented unique problems of its own. Nevertheless, her unwavering tenacity was recognized when she was awarded the 1964 Nobel Prize in Chemistry. Her work to develop X-ray crystallography had been acknowledged as truly pioneering, and the system became a widely used tool, critical in later determining the structures of many biological molecules where knowledge of structure is

'Plots of final structure Penicillin', graph of chemical structure by Hodgkin, 1946. Oxford, Bodleian Library MS. Eng. c. 5603/15. Hodgkin won her Nobel Prize for Chemistry in 1964, 'for her determinations by X-ray techniques of important biochemical substances'.

fundamental to an understanding of function. By giving a picture of how the atoms fitted together in the molecule, Hodgkin made an invaluable contribution to science and gave biology a precious roadmap of understanding.

At her memorial service at the University Church in Oxford on 4 March 1995, the molecular biologist Max Perutz encapsulated her life: 'There was a magic about her person. She had no enemies, not even among those whose scientific theories she demolished or whose political views she opposed…It was marvellous to have her drop in on you in the lab, like the spring. Dorothy will be remembered as a great chemist, a saintly, tolerant and gentle lover of people and a devoted protagonist of peace.'[37] Remarkably, she remains the only British woman to have won a science Nobel Prize.

Dorothy Hodgkin letter to Thomas, 29 September 1943, 'a very exciting day the first half of penicillin has been synthesized'. Oxford, Bodleian Library, MS. Eng. c. 7934/8. ©The estate of Dorothy Crowfoot Hodgkin

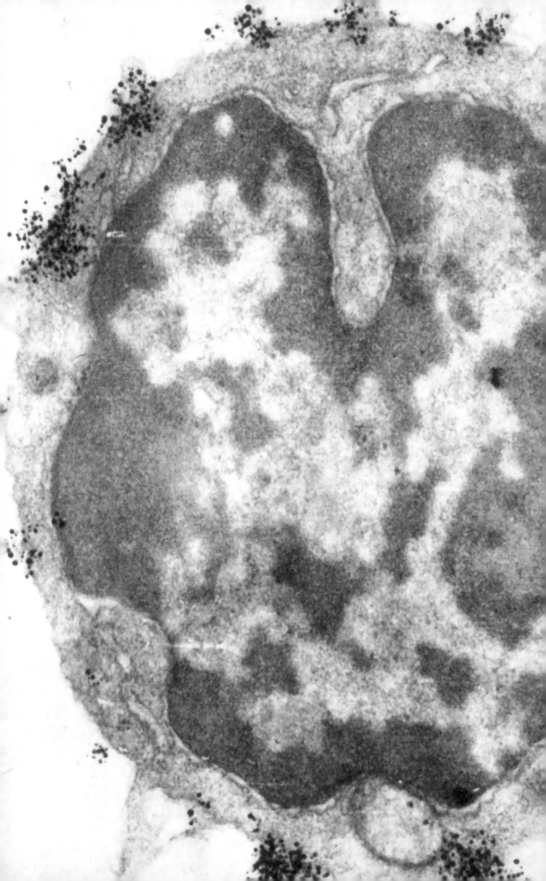

James Gowans

'The mysterious lymphocyte'

Uncovering the role of the mysterious lymphocyte – a white blood cell – was one of the landmark discoveries in post-war medicine. Not only did it illuminate 'one of the most humiliating and disgraceful gaps in all medical knowledge'; it also ushered in the new era of immunology.[38] In 1953, James (Jim) Gowans, having spent a sabbatical at the Pasteur Institute in Paris – where he gained an interest in infection and immunity – returned to Oxford and to his mentor at the William Dunn School of Pathology, Howard Florey. It was Florey who suggested to Gowans that the life history of the small lymphocyte, a major component of lymphoid tissue which accumulated, often in large numbers, in a variety of pathological lesions, might prove a fruitful area for study. He set the young physiologist off on his research mission with a customary lack of expectation: 'The role of the lymphocyte has blunted the wits of a whole generation of workers in my lab Gowans, and I don't see why you should be excused from the same fate.'[39]

By tracing the route of the blood cells in rats by using radioactive labelling, Gowans soon showed that the small lymphocyte continuously recirculated from the blood to the lymph and back again into the blood. With this telling experiment, Gowans had solved the mystery of where the cells went, so the next question was: what did they do? With the help of Peter Medawar, the renowned British immunologist, Gowans then discovered that lymph nodes could transfer immunity, for instance in

A lymphocyte is a white cell in the vertebrate immune system. Lymphocytes can be identified by their relatively large nucleus. Image courtesy of Simon Hunt and James Gowans.

the case of skin grafts, in a process known as adoptive transfer.[40] Thus immunity and immune response resided in the lymphoid tissue. Although the lymphocyte is a small and unprepossessing-looking cell, Gowans had proved that it was the seat of immunological reaction.

The immune system is the body's defence mechanism against infectious organisms. It was soon recognized that there are two main classes of lymphocytes, 'B' cells and 'T' cells, which, along with antibodies, help to bind to antigens. Gowans's revolutionary insight, together with collaborative research in New York with Jonathan Uhr, showed that lymphocytes were the locus of immunological cell-based memory. Once produced, lymphocytes remain in a person's body, so that if the same antigen is presented to the immune system again, the lymphocytes are already there to do their job. In this way, if a person contracts chickenpox it is unlikely to recur. Without the lymphocyte we would therefore succumb to infectious diseases and die young. The use of highly successful vaccines depends on stimulating lymphocytes into immunological action. Alas, this vast microscopic defence mechanism also presents biological disadvantages. Increasingly, as populations grow older, more people require transplants, which cannot be done without immunosuppressing drugs. Suppressing immunity is a hazardous undertaking and leaves people vulnerable to debilitating infections normally held in check by lymphocytes.

In 1962, Irving Weissman, a medical student at Stanford, California, was at a meeting of the New York Academy of Sciences when Gowans gave a historic talk on his work: 'For me that moment was a flash of clarity that this was a quantum jump from implication by morphology to definition by physiological *in vivo* experimentation. I joined the audience in a standing ovation, the only one I have ever seen for a scientific talk.'[41]

The three major types of lymphocyte are T cells, B cells and natural killer (NK) cells. T cells and B cells are the major cellular components of adaptive immune response. Image courtesy of Simon Hunt.

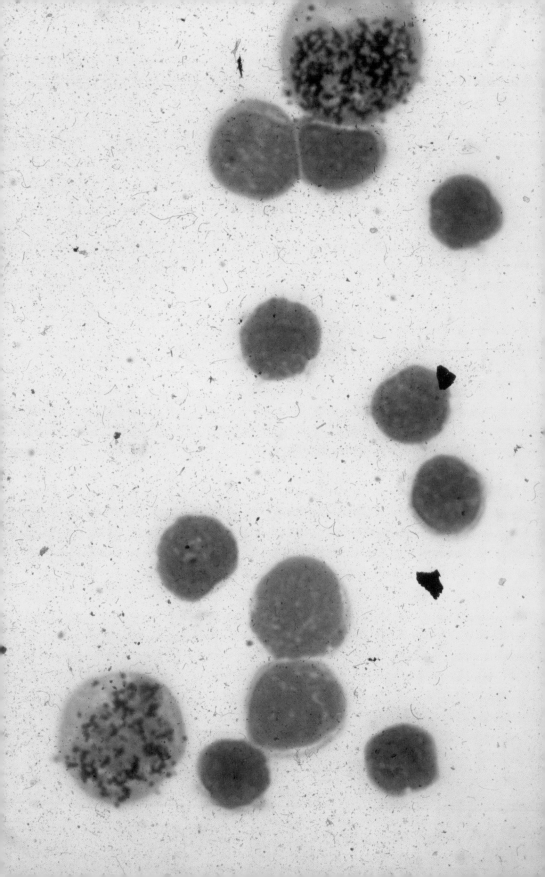

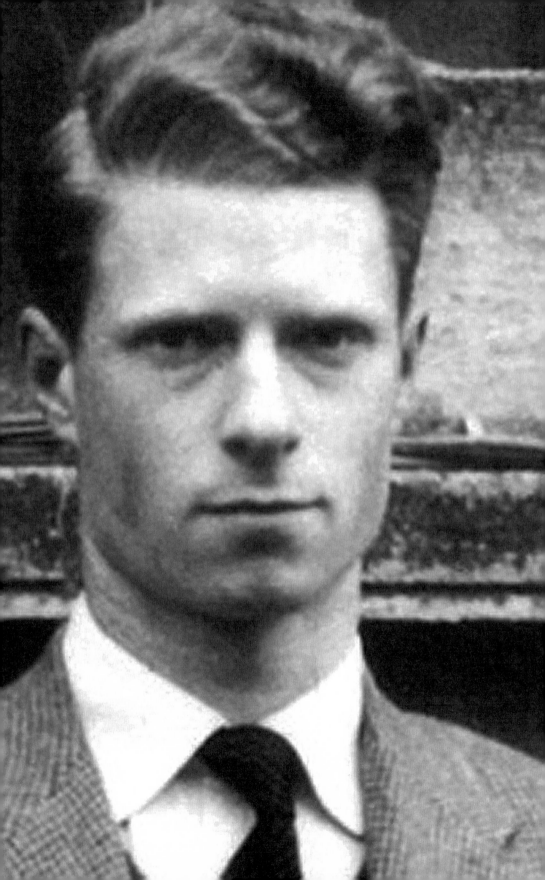

The cloning era

Oxford science's association with the cell, which began with Robert Hooke in the seventeenth century, was recognised and celebrated in 2012 when Sir John Gurdon was awarded the Nobel Prize in Physiology or Medicine for his work on reprogramming ordinary cells into immature stem cells. He shared the prize with Shinya Yamanaka for the discovery that mature, specialized cells can be reprogrammed to become immature cells capable of developing into all tissues in the body. 'Their findings', the Nobel Assembly at the Karolinska Institute said of Gurdon and Yamanaka, 'have revolutionised our understanding of how cells and organisms develop.'[42]

John Gurdon spent most of his scientific career in Cambridge, but it was his work carried out in Oxford that won him the Nobel Prize. He started his DPhil project in 1956 in the Zoology Department, supervised by Mikhail (Mischa) Fischberg, a noted embryologist. Using a technique known as nuclear transfer (a form of cloning), he showed that differentiation and development are reversible. This was very important because it had been universally believed that adulthood was a fixed end point for cellular function.[43] In his classic experiment, published in 1962, he replaced the immature cell nucleus in an egg cell of a frog – the South African clawed frog – with the nucleus of a mature intestinal cell.[44] The modified egg cell developed into a normal tadpole and went on to live a normal frog life-span. One of Gurdon's colleagues in the lab, Tom

John Gurdon. Department of Zoology, University of Oxford, 1958. Photograph: photographers workshop.com.

Elsdale, wrote: 'He showed great skill and persistence using the technique and he was the one who got the results with it.'[45]

Gurdon took his undergraduate degree at Christ Church, initially studying Classics but switching to Zoology. He received his doctorate from Oxford in 1960 and was a postdoctoral fellow at the California Institute of Technology before returning to Oxford as an assistant lecturer in 1962. A decade later, he became the Professor of Cell Biology at Cambridge University. While in Oxford, Gurdon held the Beit Fellowship, a scheme specifically to support the work of young scientists – seven of the holders of this award have won Nobel Prizes.[46] A striking feature of John Gurdon's Nobel Prize is that it was awarded half a century after the groundbreaking work was carried out, in tandem with Yamanaka's more recent and related findings. Perhaps it was a combination of events which finally brought the global recognition that many in the field felt was long overdue. Stem cells are certainly scientifically in vogue, with departments blossoming in Cambridge and Newcastle which aim to translate research into clinical practice in the near future.

Professor Chris Graham of the University of Oxford's Department of Zoology – and one of John Gurdon's first research students – is in no doubt of his friend's contribution to scientific knowledge. 'He showed that you could take several nuclei from one individual and produce genetically identical animals – that was his great achievement. People had talked about cloning a good deal but with John Gurdon's work, it became a reality.'[47]

Cloning apparatus (reconstruction) used by John Gurdon during the 1960s, comprising a microscope and tools for egg cell manipulation. Image courtesy of Chris Graham, Department of Zoology, University of Oxford. Photograph: photographers workshop.com.

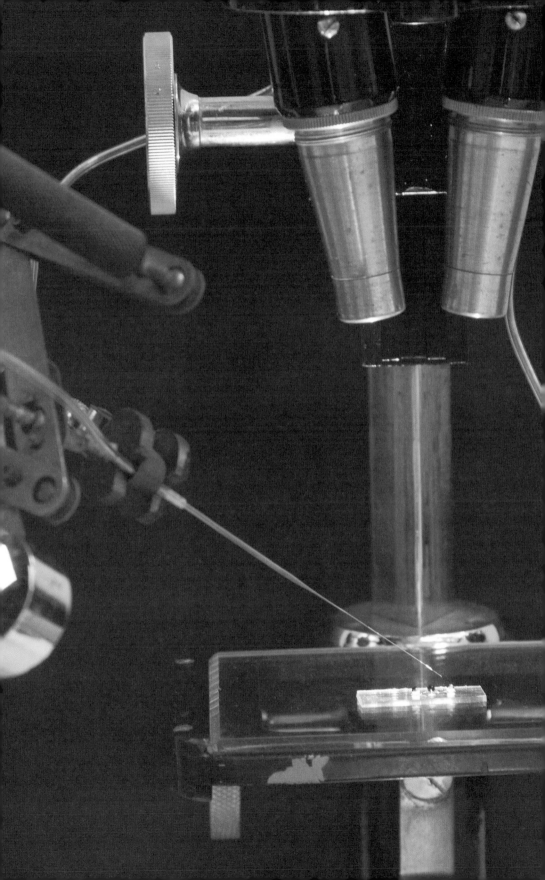

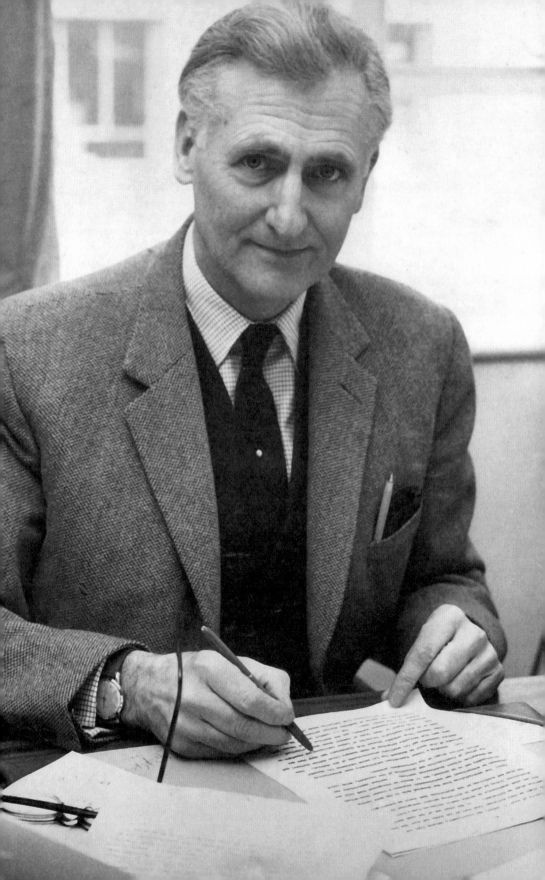

Epidemiological science

In 1950, when Richard Doll and his mentor, the medical statistician Bradford Hill, demonstrated that smoking was 'a cause and an important cause' of the rapidly increasing epidemic of lung cancer in Britain, his path in life was set. Adapting the old science of epidemiology, which had evolved in the nineteenth century to identify the causes of infectious disease, Doll expanded the discipline to discover the causes of the devastating diseases of modernity: strokes, heart attacks and, in particular, cancer. Uncovering the dangers of tobacco and showing the benefits of quitting to educationalists, politicians and the public formed a major part of Doll's scientific career. His approach was heavily reliant on the science of statistics, rather than of the stethoscope, yet his belief in statistical evidence was firmly rooted in its efficacy for the common good. In October 1951, Doll and Hill sent a short questionnaire to every doctor in Britain: the study gradually evolved into the first major prospective investigation of the links between smoking and death anywhere in the world. Doll's research proved the benefits of quitting and the resulting decline in lung cancer, heart attack and other smoking-related diseases.

Doll was an inspiring scientific investigator and he attracted to Oxford some of the most able in the field. By learning at first hand from the most accomplished cancer epidemiologist of the twentieth century, his disciples have gone on to expand the frontiers of the field, to the benefit of the health of the global population. His

Richard Doll c. 1960. More than any other physician, Doll became the world leader in the study of the health effects of smoking. Image courtesy of Doll's family.

career in Oxford will be remembered for three lasting achievements: developing the Oxford Medical School into one of the most prestigious in the world, founding Green College (now Green Templeton) and his own scientific work. During his tenure as the twenty-seventh Regius Professor of Medicine, he negotiated finance for five new chairs at the Medical School: clinical biochemistry, morbid anatomy, paediatrics, clinical biochemistry and social medicine. Within a short period of time, the Medical School was admitting one hundred students per year and, as the *Oxford Medical Gazette* reported, the new chairs were 'an indispensable part of the planned expansion'.[48] Green College as an institution focusing on medicine became an enduring success story. The college opened on 1 September 1979. In 1A Observatory Street, the Warden's home, over breakfast, Richard and his wife Joan would study photographs of the college's students so that they could greet them on first-name terms.

Doll never quite retired – his Indian summer of scientific study reached its peak with the publication on 26 June 2004 of fifty years' worth of observation on the smoking habits of male British doctors. On his ninety-second birthday that year, together with his great friend and scientific collaborator Sir Richard Peto, Doll gave a talk to a packed meeting of doctors in the lecture theatre of the John Radcliffe Hospital. Both men were relaxed and comfortable with an audience who had come to recognize the power and necessity of statistics to clinical research and hence to clinical practice. Doll sought to understand the world and to help people enjoy their lives, free from the unnecessary burden of avoidable disease. His work caused a revolution and changed the health of the nation. Knowledge that quitting smoking could have such a dramatic effect on death rates would, in time, advance public health medicine as profoundly as the introduction of inoculation or the therapeutic application

Original graph of smoking vs non-smoking mortality rates, later published in a *British Medical Journal* article, 26 June 2004, on the fiftieth anniversary of the first study of the smoking habits of male British doctors. Image courtesy of Jill Boreham and the Clinical Trials Studies Unit, Oxford.

of penicillin. A medical pioneer in the great tradition of Oxford experimental science, Doll represented the ultimate in dedication, perseverance and integrity.

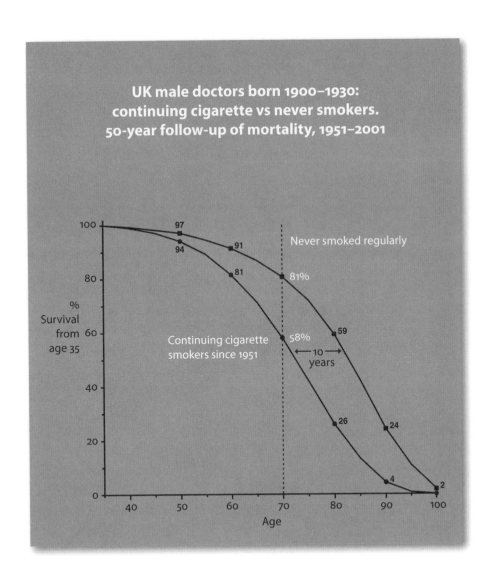

UK male doctors born 1900–1930: continuing cigarette vs never smokers. 50-year follow-up of mortality, 1951–2001

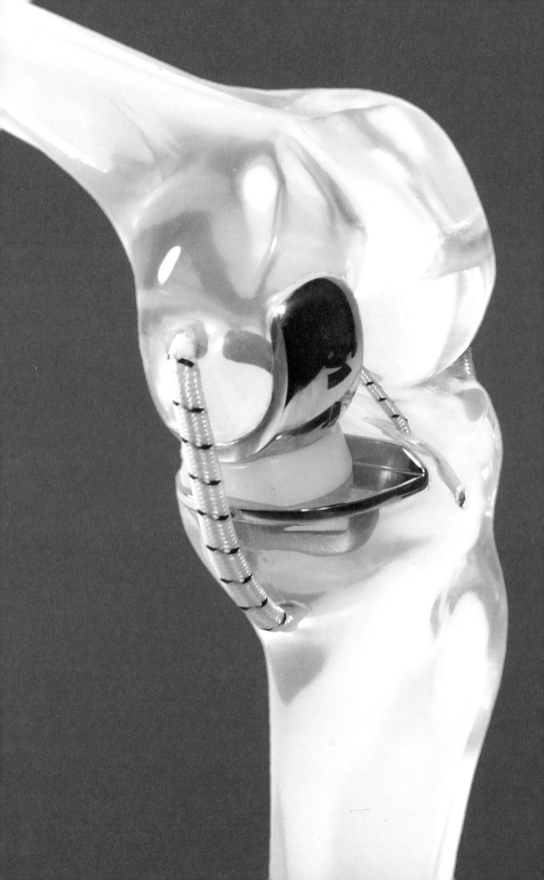

The Oxford Knee

A revolution in joint replacement

For scientists, serendipitous events or the play of chance can influence the direction of careers and, on occasion, plot the route of entirely new ones. In 1964, John O'Connor, a young Irish engineer, took up a college fellowship in engineering at St Peter's College, Oxford. Two years later, the *University Gazette* announced that he had secured his first major research grant to examine: 'the fatigue strength of clamped joints'.[49] Shortly afterwards, he received a phone call from John Goodfellow, an orthopaedic surgeon at the Nuffield Orthopaedic Centre, Headington, Oxford: 'I see you're interested in clamped joints, whatever they are? Could you possibly be interested in hip joints?'[50] O'Connor was indeed interested, and together they began a study of load bearing in the human hip.

By the end of the decade, their unique and unlikely collaboration had led them from investigating the hip to the immensely more complicated human knee joint. In the 1970s, knee replacement was very uncommon, yet the need for such operations was high: osteoarthritis of the knee was, and still is, one of the most common causes of a painful loss of mobility in middle-aged and elderly people, and is the main driver of knee replacement surgery. Using mathematical modelling while seeking guidance from the anatomical drawings of Leonardo da Vinci, the men set about inventing an alternative to a total knee replacement. The pioneering work began in the lab and was then transferred to the operating theatre.

Perspex model of the Oxford Knee – showing unicompartmental replacement, with a plastic analogue of the natural meniscus interposed between metal components attached to the bones. The design of the articular surfaces of the Oxford Knee has not changed since its first implantation in 1976.

For O'Connor, the task was intellectually compelling: 'the menisci and cartilage form mobile sockets between bones, and then it came to us, if nature needs to use mobile menisci in its knee, why not in an artificial knee? We made up bits and pieces in the lab and eventually got as close to a replica of a human knee as possible made out of metal and plastic.'[51] Their invention, named the 'Oxford Knee', was designed to replace only the damaged half of the knee, thereby avoiding many of the inescapable shortcomings of a total replacement. In the latter operation, the anterior cruciate ligament, if still intact, is severed, allowing direct and easier access to the knee joint, which makes the entire operation relatively straightforward. One of the recognized advantages of the Oxford Knee, however, is that it is far less invasive, only replacing the worn surfaces rather than the whole joint, thus retaining all of the ligaments, which are important for optimal post-operative recovery and mobility.

In 1976, John Goodfellow carried out the first Oxford Knee operation. In September 2011, a thirty-fifth anniversary celebration of this pioneering event was held at Keble College, Oxford. While initially the procedure was viewed with scepticism within the orthopaedic surgical community, Professor David Murray and Mr Chris Dodd, who developed the minimally invasive operation technique and associated surgical instruments, have since 1998, taught more than 10,000 surgeons worldwide how to identify appropriate patients and how to perform the operation. The implantable components and surgical instruments are made by Biomet UK Ltd in Swindon and Bridgend. Today the vast majority of Oxford Knee operations are carried out far away from the city that through a combination of nurture, nature and serendipity was responsible for its invention.

A patient's knee before closure, with the implant clearly visible. Image courtesy of David Murray and John O'Connor.

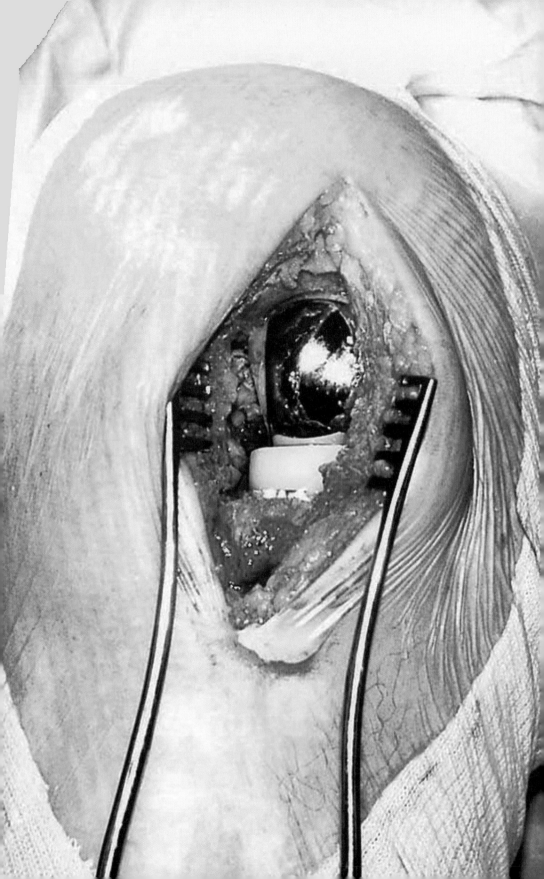

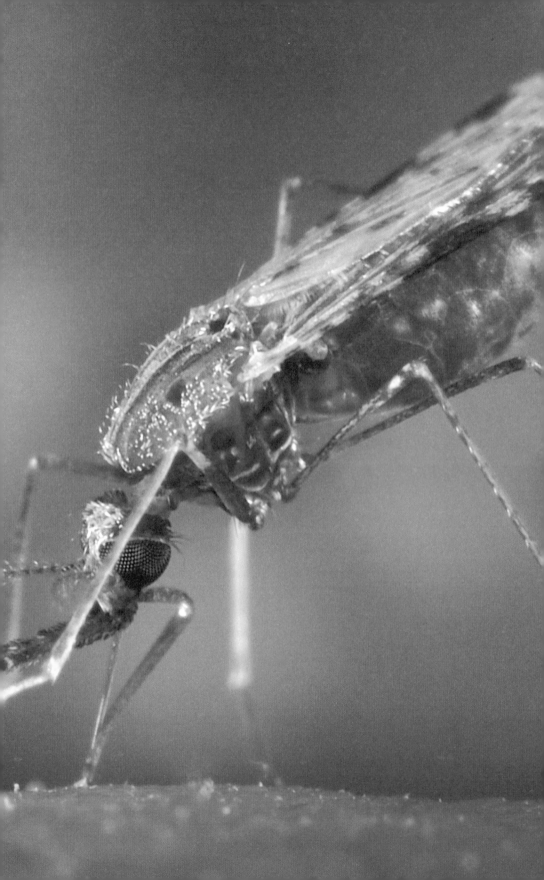

Tropical Medicine

Transnational partnerships in the developing world

Throughout the developing world, millions of people die annually from the preventable diseases that have been eliminated in the richer countries of the northern hemisphere. This invidious and avoidable tragedy was the incentive for David Weatherall, the Nuffield Professor of Medicine, to accept an invitation in 1978 from the Rockefeller Foundation in New York to establish the 'Great Neglected Diseases of Mankind' programme, which would create a network of high-quality investigators in the field. Also invited was the then director of the Wellcome Trust, Peter Williams. Famously, over a particularly good bottle of Scotch, one of the greatest programmes in the long history of Oxford medicine was formulated. Both men had lived and worked in the tropics and shared a vision for medicine in a post-colonial world. Their strategy was to alter the concept of tropical medicine to 'medicine in the tropics'. They believed that forming genuine partnerships between Oxford medicine and a centre in the developing world, sustained by long-term funding, would be the best way forward.[52]

As a result, the Mahidol-Oxford-Wellcome Unit opened in Bangkok, Thailand, in May 1979, with David Warrell as director. A year later, Nick White, a specialist in infectious diseases, joined the unit. Their collective determination, scientific originality and steadfastness laid the foundations for the model of medicine in the tropics at both basic and applied levels. White has

Anopheles mosquito. Malaria is transmitted among humans by female mosquitoes of the genus *Anopheles*. Image courtesy of the Liverpool School of Tropical Medicine.

now spent over thirty years in Thailand and his work, especially in the field of malaria control, has transformed our understanding of the disease.[53] Using clinical trials and meta-analysis, White and his colleagues showed unequivocally that the drug parenteral artesunate should replace quinine as the treatment of choice for severe falciparum malaria worldwide.[54]

The success of the Bangkok unit inspired other physician-scientists from Oxford to carry out similar research. Africa, the world's most malarious continent, was a natural choice. In 1987, Kevin Marsh visited Kilifi on the Kenyan coast, an area particularly debilitated by the disease. He recognised that the region offered great possibilities for an integrated programme of research on malaria that linked scientific, clinical and epidemiological approaches. In 1989, the Kenya Medical Research Institute (KEMRI)–Oxford–Wellcome Programme began its work, and under Marsh has grown into the most effective and prestigious research institution in Africa. Its state-of-the-art laboratory is home to 800 staff and trains African scientists for careers in disease control. Through basic research, bed-net

Map of the distribution of malaria. Despite massive efforts to eradicate the disease, it remains a major public health problem in poorer tropical regions. Image courtesy of Catherine Moyes, Department of Zoology, University of Oxford.

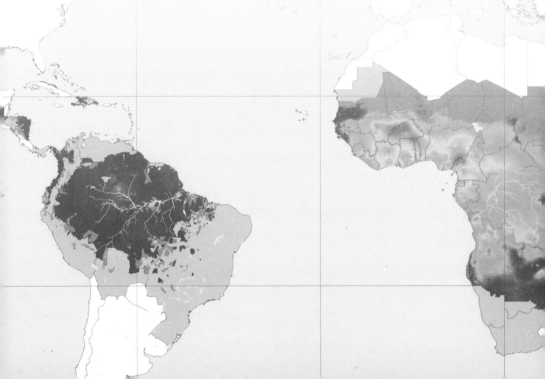

programmes and integrated public health measures, malaria, which was once at the apex of the 'great neglected diseases', is now decreasing in many countries across Asia and Africa.

Tropical medicine is one of Oxford's great achievements. Weatherall, the architect of the idea, is in no doubt that many of the physicians who decided to work in the tropics were motivated, in some part, by altruism and wanted to free people from the burden of avoidable diseases. This dedication is symptomatic of the ethos that has guided tropical medicine for more than thirty years. Today, Oxford medicine has a presence in India, China, Southeast Asia, Africa and South America. It is one of the University of Oxford's major contemporary achievements and hascontributed to the university's global presence and celebrated reputation for excellence. In 2012, the *Times Higher Education* evaluation of world university rankings placed Oxford medicine at the top of the list: 'it is in medical research where Oxford really stands out, bolstered by the longest cluster of overseas research activity across the entire university – the Africa and Asia Tropical Medicine network.'[55]

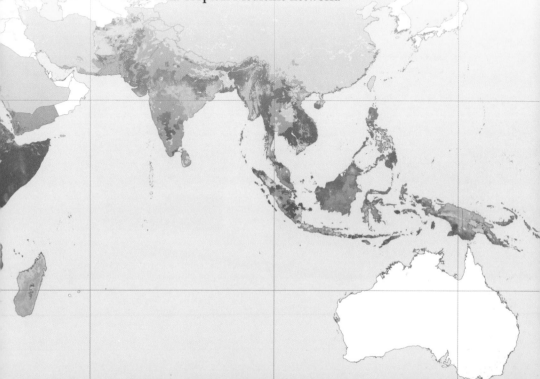

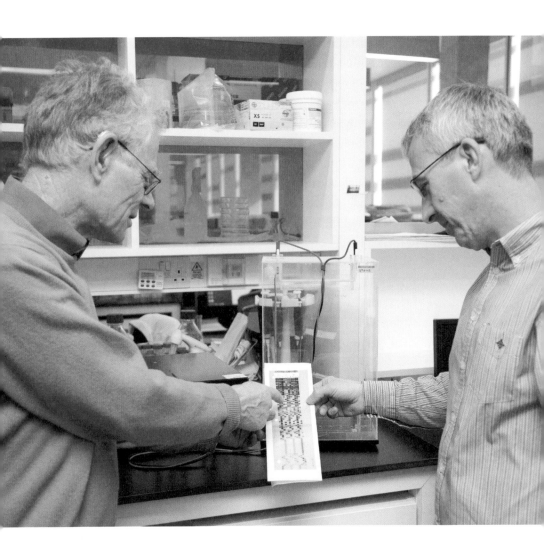

Haemophilia

Inherited blood diseases

Charles Darwin had been fascinated with the concept of disease inheritance, while Archibald Garrod, Regius Professor of Medicine at Oxford in the 1920s, had concluded that some diseases arose out of an inborn 'error of metabolism' which was congenital.[56] Basic science, clinical research and practical medicine came together in the second half of the twentieth century in the form of genetics. The effects were life-changing, and explained for the first time how diseases could be genetically inherited. One great mystery to be unravelled by genetics was the cause of haemophilia, a rare and hereditary blood coagulation disorder caused by a mutation in the Factor VIII gene (classic haemophilia) or the Factor IX gene (Christmas disease). There are thus two forms of inherited haemophilia, both determined by genes located on the X chromosome and affecting males and not females, who instead act as carriers. Although unaffected, females can transmit their inborn error to the next generation and produce male haemophiliacs.

The disease epitomizes the profound effect that such ailments can play on the course of history. Queen Victoria was a carrier of the disease because of a mutation in the Factor IX gene, and due to the close dynastic relations of the major European royal families, haemophilia spread to the Russian and Spanish royal families through marriage to Queen Victoria's 'carrier' daughters. As a consequence, haemophilia became known popularly as 'the royal disease'. The Romanov

George Brownlee and Ervin Fodor at the Dunn School of Pathology, Oxford, discussing an archive autoradiograph of a polyacrylamide separation of radioactively labelled DNA sequenced by the Sanger dideoxy chain termination method. This method was routine in the 1980s and 1990s. Photograph: photographers workshop.com.

dynasty were also known carriers of a rare strain of haemophilia B. Today, haemophilia is no longer a death sentence and can be successfully treated, primarily due to the ingenuity and application of Oxford scientists.

Gwyn Macfarlane (1907–1987) arrived at the Radcliffe Infirmary in 1940. Within a decade he was able to isolate the anti-haemophilic factor, Factor VIII. This led the way to the possibility of treating haemophiliacs and enabling surgery to be carried out without fatal blood loss. Oxford was soon recognized as one of the world's leading centres for the investigation of haemophilia, thanks partially to what was perhaps Macfarlane's greatest contribution to modern medicine: the deciphering of the enzyme cascade process of blood coagulation. The disease resulting from lack of Factor IX also became known as 'Christmas disease', named after Stephen Christmas, one of Macfarlane's patients in Oxford.[57] The introduction of replacement therapy was to transform life for the haemophiliac. For Macfarlane, who started out in the field of coagulation when so little was known, to have seen it through almost to the recombinant DNA era was a remarkable achievement.

Further developments occurred in the 1970s. David Weatherall was appointed the Nuffield Professor of Medicine in 1974. With him came the application of molecular insights into blood-borne diseases. In 1978, the molecular biologist George Brownlee took up his post in Oxford, after spending his formative scientific years working with Fred Sanger in Cambridge at the Medical Research Council's Laboratory of Molecular Biology. His arrival heralded a groundbreaking shift: scientific analysis had moved from organs, to tissues, to cells, to molecules. Visitors to Brownlee's laboratory watched as pioneering new sequencing techniques were developed, which had practical application in the science of disease inheritance. Brownlee was interested in pure research but he also recognized the usefulness of being able to apply molecular techniques to addressing human diseases, particularly blood diseases. 'I knew David Weatherall was working on haemoglobin and thalassemias, so I didn't want to go there, but haemophilia B was interesting and it was a conscious decision on my part to investigate it – it was feasible.'[58] Within eighteen months, Brownlee and his team had made a breakthrough that could not have come at a more dramatic time. The HIV/AIDS virus was infecting haemophiliacs, and so a Factor IX preparation derived from a source other than human blood was urgently required. Beginning his research on rats, Brownlee successfully cloned and expressed human clotting Factor IX, providing a recombinant source of this protein for haemophilia B patients who had previously relied on the hazardous blood-derived product.[59] Brownlee's research put an end to the so-called 'motorway of infection' that had such tragic consequences for haemophiliacs. Collectively, the work undertaken in Oxford transformed the lives of haemophiliacs, previously fearful of injury and doomed to an early death, to ones similar to those whose genes had not denied them innate clotting agents.

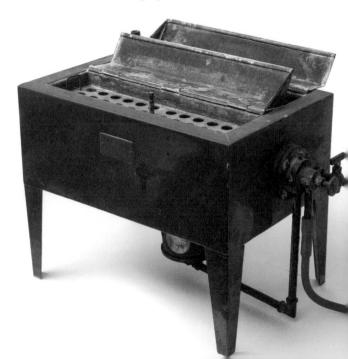

Brass water bath, heated by a gas burner, used to measure the clotting time of blood, *circa* 1960. At the time Professor Gwyn Macfarlane FRS was the director of the MRC's Blood Coagulation Research Unit. Image courtesy of the Churchill Hospital, Oxford. Photograph: photographers workshop.com.

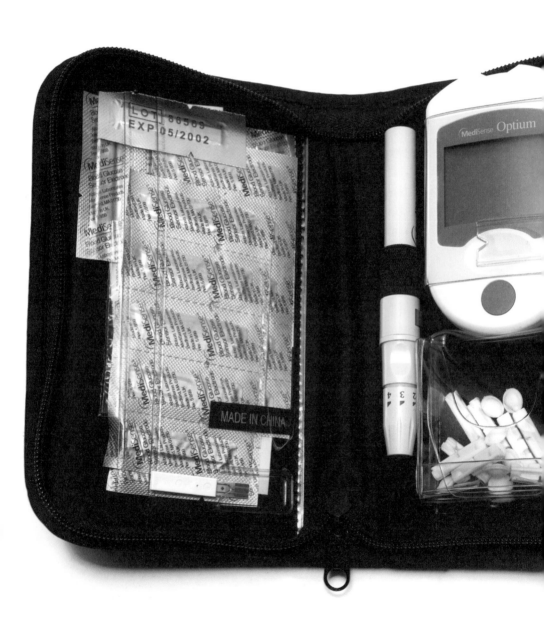

The Glucose Biosensor

Diabetes in the modern world

We all need insulin to live – it helps to regulate our metabolism and prevents potentially dangerous levels of glucose from building up in the bloodstream. However, when the body's control of insulin levels fails, diabetes mellitus – or simply diabetes, as it is better known – can result. The high blood sugar levels characterized by diabetes not only lead to a variety of symptoms including weight loss, abdominal pain and blurred vision, but also significantly increase the risk of long-term complications, most notably cardiovascular disease. Diabetes now poses a considerable threat: cases are increasing rapidly throughout the world, while over 3 million people in Britain alone have been diagnosed with the disease.[60]

The milestone discovery of the glucose electrode by Oxford University's Allen Hill and co-workers in 1982 has had a substantial and transformative effect on the lives of millions of diabetes sufferers. Hill's invention, which monitors the amount of sugar in a blood sample, allows diabetics to manage their condition easily, free from anxiety, thanks to the accurate, discreet and convenient biosensor.

The origin of Hill's discovery may have emanated from his family history: his father had died as a type 2 diabetic, and his Hungarian wife's family members had also been diagnosed with the disease.[61] Three other elements were indispensable to his pioneering work: time, inspirational colleagues and financial support. In 1976–77, Hill was Senior Proctor of the University.

The glucose biosensor has evolved into an easy-to-use and indispensable device for measuring blood glucose for millions of people with diabetes around the world. 27 billion blood glucose test strips have been sold since their invention in Oxford in the 1980s.

His precious Wednesday afternoons were free from University duties, allowing him 'the opportunity to have interactions with my research group … invaluable for building and thinking.'[62] Initially, most of Hill's group worked on electrochemistry, nuclear magnetic resonance and electron transfer to redox-active enzymes, and by the 1980s these experiments had yielded an important breakthrough. Hill and his colleague Graham Davis had already made successful studies of the electrochemistry of enzymes, but their systems to test chemical reactions were very sensitive to oxygen. With the help of a third scientist, Tony Cass, the team discovered that a compound, ferrocene, when associated with the necessary enzymes, would render the interference of oxygen in their experiments obsolete. When they further demonstrated that such enzyme reactions could take place in blood, the foundations for the glucose sensor had been formed.

Hill had envisaged a device to test blood samples as early as 1977. Now, together with his colleagues, he developed the technology to determine blood glucose levels rapidly, precisely and economically, from a single drop of blood placed on the testing strip of a sensor. The team travelled the country seeking financial support to bring their design into mass production. Although the scientific community was supportive, those with control over money were less forthcoming. Nevertheless, by the end of the 1980s the company MediSense had been established to manufacture the new sensor, which entered the market in 1989. The initial pen-like device was superseded by a more successful 'credit card' design, which gives faster results via a more user-friendly display, and is now instantly recognizable to diabetics around the world.

For their collective dedication, the Oxford researchers have been commemorated with a blue plaque at the Inorganic Chemistry Laboratory, Oxford, which aptly

The National Chemical
Landmark blue plaque
presented by the Royal
Society of Chemistry, on
the wall of the Oxford
laboratory where Hill,
Cass and Davis carried
out their celebrated
work in the 1980s. Image
courtesy of the Inorganic
Chemistry Laboratory,
University of Oxford.

summarizes their work: 'In this laboratory on 20 July 1982, Allen Hill, Tony Cass and Graham Davis made the crucial discovery which led to the development of a unique electronic blood sensor now used by millions of diabetics worldwide.'

RSC | Advancing the Chemical Sciences

National Chemical Landmark

Glucose Sensor

In this laboratory on 20th July 1982, Allen Hill, Tony Cass and Graham Davis made the crucial discovery which led to the development of a unique electronic blood glucose sensor now used by millions of diabetics worldwide.

16 July 2012

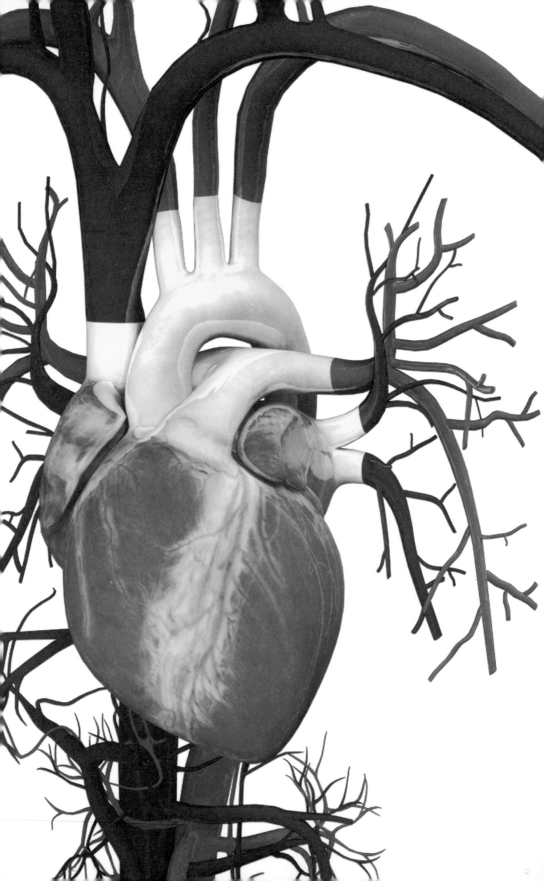

The mega-trial breakthrough

The ISIS-2 randomized controlled trial was the culmination of a statistical hypothesis that Professor Richard Peto had advocated as a way to impact on the big killers facing humanity.[63] Peto and his colleague Rory Collins used epidemiological science to give clinicians dealing with patients in hospitals the most reliable information about the best treatments to help reduce mortality levels. The ISIS-2 trial, with its very large patient cohort, geographical spread and dramatic findings, not only helped to change clinical practice and reduce deaths; it also became a model for the design of randomized control trials of the future. Until the 1980s, most clinical trials were hopelessly inadequate in size – they did not have the power to test reliably the value of a moderate but worthwhile treatment in many common conditions. What Collins and his colleagues wanted to investigate was the efficacy of blood clot-busting drugs (thrombolytics) in patients who had suffered a heart attack. Prior to the ISIS-2 trial, when a patient came into a cardiac unit they were given pain killers, and doctors waited to see if a lethal arrhythmia followed. If it did, they would attempt to electrically shock the patient out of the potentially fatal condition. There was little else to the treatment. Unlike previous randomized controlled trials, the ISIS 2 trial was a far more ambitious undertaking. Beautifully designed, it tested the effects of intravenous streptokinase, oral aspirin, both, or neither, among 17,187 cases of suspected acute myocardial infarction (heart

3D illustration of the human heart and circulatory system. Image courtesy of Bryan Brandenburg.

attack).[64] It involved 417 hospitals with a 'blind' treatment regime – cardiologists did not know if they were giving the patient an active drug or a placebo, which removed the subjectivity of the clinician from the experiment. The pharmaceuticals company Behringwerke, a subsidiary of Hoechst, financed the trial at a cost of $2 million, and was persuaded to 'factor in' aspirin, even though at the time their drug package carried a warning of the dangers of combining streptokinase and aspirin.[65]

The trial took three years to complete. When the results were published in *The Lancet* in 1988, they were so impressive and compelling as to change medical practice. Streptokinase reduced mortality by 20–25 per cent, aspirin by another 25 per cent, and when taken together these treatments reduced mortality by half. The difference between having a heart attack thirty years ago and now is that the mortality risk is about one-third of what it was then. These effects on mortality were only discernible because the trial was so large, giving unequivocal results. There was no need for complex mathematical analysis: the findings were indisputable. As a renowned advocate of big numbers, Rory Collins draws an intriguing analogy: 'It is like a microscope – you're able to see something that you didn't know exists and you're able to understand that it is important.'[66] The ISIS-2 trial undoubtedly contributed greatly to the treatment of cardiac disease, yet its more fundamental legacy is in showing the value of large-scale randomized controlled trials, which are now the benchmark of medical research.

Original graph showing the effects of streptokinase and aspirin on mortality rates as part of the ISIS-2 trial. Later published in *The Lancet* 2, 1988. Image courtesy of Sarah Parish and the Clinical Trials Studies Unit, Oxford.

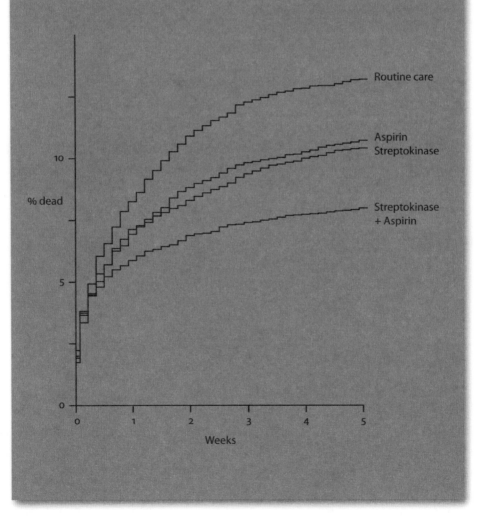

Lives saved in ISIS-2 among 17187 heart attack patients who would not normally have received streptokinase or aspirin, divided at random into 4 similar groups to get aspirin only, streptokinase only, both or neither.

Any doctor who delieved that a particular patient should be given either treatment gave it, and did not include the patient in ISIS-2

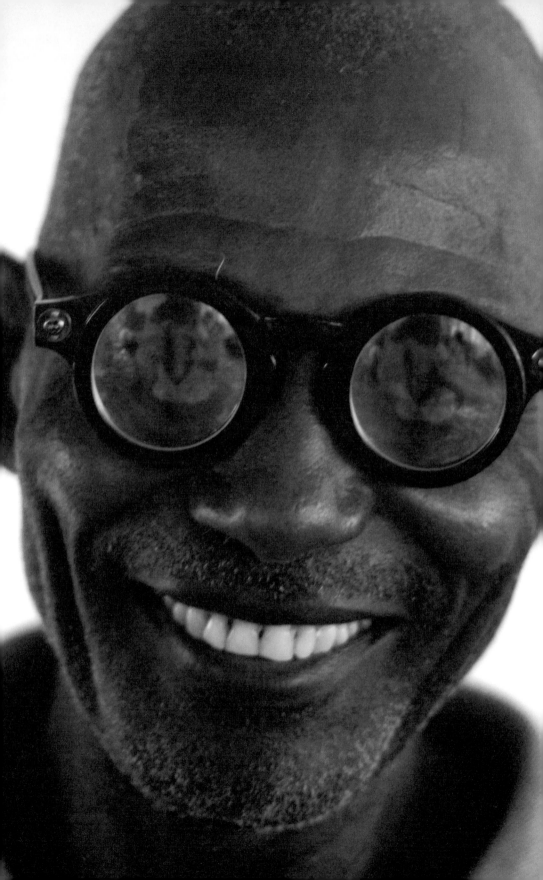

Joshua Silver

Self-refraction eyeglasses

A simple idea can change health care forever, and
Oxford has an impressive tradition of innovation that
has transformed global health. Joshua Silver is part of
this celebrated history: an atomic physicist-turned-vision
scientist, Silver's ambition is to improve the eyesight of
one billion of the world's poorest people.

In Britain, a simple trip to the optician can provide
a prescription for corrective eyeglasses. If you wear
glasses or contact lenses, you know that being able to
see precisely is a vital part of our everyday existence
– it affects our education, our work and our health.
According to the World Health Organization, however,
over one billion people would benefit from glasses but
do not have access to them. As a case in point, in Britain
there is one optometrist for every 4,500 people, but
in some parts of sub-Saharan Africa the ratio can be
1:1,000,000. Even if trained opticians worked for free in
the Third World, this would not be the answer to what is
a tremendous and growing need.

Answering this great need is Joshua Silver's original,
innovative and simple invention. In March 1985, Silver
was discussing with a colleague if it might be possible to
make a lens of variable focus. Silver became interested in
variable focus lenses and first made a crude one in his lab
in March 1985. As he considered the problem, he realized
that a technique he had used since the 1970s to seal and
stretch plastic membranes could be employed to make
a fluid-filled variable focus lens of good optical quality,

A man from Liberia
wearing a pair of Adspecs
eyeglasses.
Image courtesy of the
Centre for Vision in the
Developing World.

and in May 1985 he made a new lens with which he was able to correct his own myopia with great accuracy. Silver later used this technique to create eyeglasses that enabled the wearer to set the focus themselves, using a small syringe attached to each arm of the spectacles which may be used to inflate or deflate the lenses.[67] The wearer simply adjusts a dial on the syringe to add or reduce the amount of silicone fluid in the membrane, thereby changing the power of the lens. With very little guidance, people are perfectly capable of creating glasses to their own prescription.

Silver says that he simply 'likes doing things out of curiosity'. This motivation has seen trials of his eyeglasses in countries across the world, first with adults, supported by the UK's overseas aid agency DFID, and later with myopic teenagers, supported by the World Bank.[68] Anthony Bron, the distinguished ophthalmic researcher, sees Silver's work as novel and 'highly original' with 'a potential global sight-saving impact'.[69] Meanwhile, new designs are on the way so the rather clunky and austere eyeglasses that have become so recognizable may soon be replaced by something more fashionable. Today, over 50,000 pairs of Silver's spectacles have been distributed in over fifteen countries, and this is only the beginning of his efforts to improve the eyesight of the world's poorest populations. He aims to dispense one billion pairs of the eyeglasses, which will cost about £2 each to make, by 2020.

Silver is currently the director of the Centre for Vision in the Developing World (CVDW) at Oxford University, which holds that everyone, no matter where they live, should be able to see as clearly as possible. His present focus is on making eyeglasses for myopic teenagers, as estimates suggest that over 100 million are simply unable to read the blackboard at school. Child Vision is a new initiative being launched by the

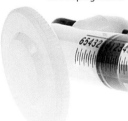

Silver's Adspecs adaptive eyeglasses – over 50,000 pairs of which are now being worn around the world. Image courtesy of the Centre for Vision in the Developing World.

CVDW and the Dow Corning Corporation; Silver hopes that by creating an awareness of the problem and enlisting the cooperation of governments, the UN and the WHO, great social progress will follow, aided by the distribution of his eyeglasses.

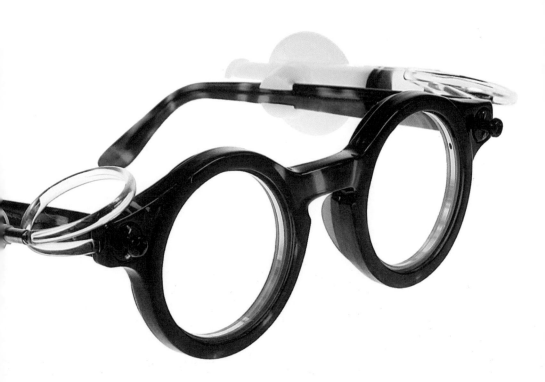

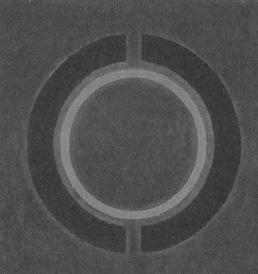
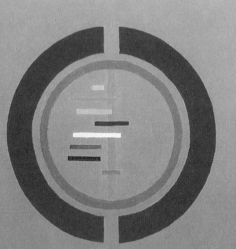
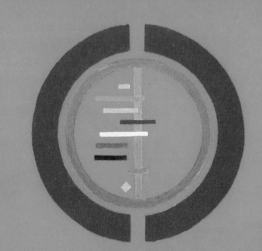

DAVID HOSTON 2.08

The Cochrane Collaboration (1993–)

Meta-analysis of medical research

One question that concerns all of us as patients is how effective a treatment is for an illness. This is the foundation upon which clinical trials are based. The aim of these controlled trials is very simple: to ensure that the comparisons we make between different treatments are as precise, as informative and as convincing as possible.[70] However, since its inception in 1993, the Cochrane Collaboration, a non-profit body which systematically organizes research information, has shown that only about 50 per cent of controlled trials are actually published, leading to a somewhat equivocal picture of what is the best care policy. One of the central roles of the Collaboration is to liberate the results of unpublished clinical trials from their neglect, with the aim of pulling together separate strands of research into a coherent, useful and reliable guide to best outcomes.

The ideological principles of the Cochrane Collaboration had been incubating in the mind of Iain Chalmers, a clinical epidemiologist, since the 1970s, when he spent two years working for the UN in Gaza. 'Some of the treatments I had been taught to give at medical school were actually harming, and sometimes killing, my patients. With the best of intentions, doctors can do harm. Everything starts from that.'[71] The idea of randomization in clinical trials and performing the statistical analysis on the results now forms an integral part of most serious medical research; yet until the Collaboration was founded there was little overarching comparative study across a range of clinical trials to compare and contrast their results. As Chalmers acknowledges, 'it was silly to try and come to a conclusion on the basis of one study, so you needed to try and get *all* of the relevant studies that had been published'.[72]

Utilizing the statistical technique of meta-analysis, Chalmers produced pioneering evidence-based results in the field of perinatal care. Meta-analysis allows researchers to combine the results of several different trials in order to provide an overview of the findings. The clarity of this analysis is reflected in the Cochrane Collaboration's logo, a graphic representation of the meta-analysis of a number of clinical trials where women who had been expected to give birth prematurely had been treated with steroids. Although individual results were inconclusive, putting together the data, symbolized in the logo by the circle, demonstrated the efficacy of the

Newborn babies and a study into their life chances were the catalyst for establishing the Cochrane Collaboration. A systematic review of an inexpensive course of corticosteroid given to women about to give birth too early reduced the odds of the babies of such women dying from the complications of immaturity by 30–50 percent. Image of sleeping newborn infant courtesy of Andrés Nieto Porras, Palma de Majorca, Spain.

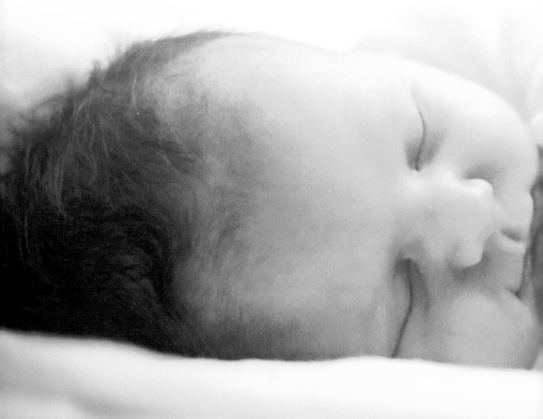

steroid treatment in reducing premature delivery. One trial alone would not give a clear picture, but when all seven trials are added together, the data is statistically significant even to the untrained eye. Until this dramatic evidence had been produced, babies were dying unnecessarily, parents were being bereaved needlessly and health services were spending money on neo-natal intensive care which was wasted.

In 1992, this breakthrough discovery led Michael Peckham, the first director of Research and Development in the NHS, to approve funding for the Cochrane Centre in Oxford, which a year later gave birth to the Cochrane Collaboration, named after Archie Cochrane, a pioneer of evidence-based medicine. Now rolled out across the globe, the Cochrane Collaboration – which started out with four employees – has a presence in one hundred countries, with over 28,000 volunteers contributing to its dedicated aim of making up-to-date, accurate information about the effects of health care readily available worldwide.

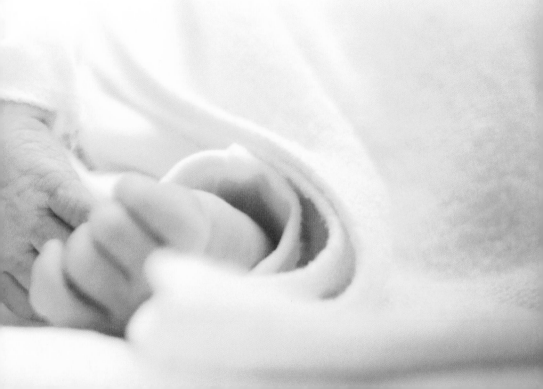

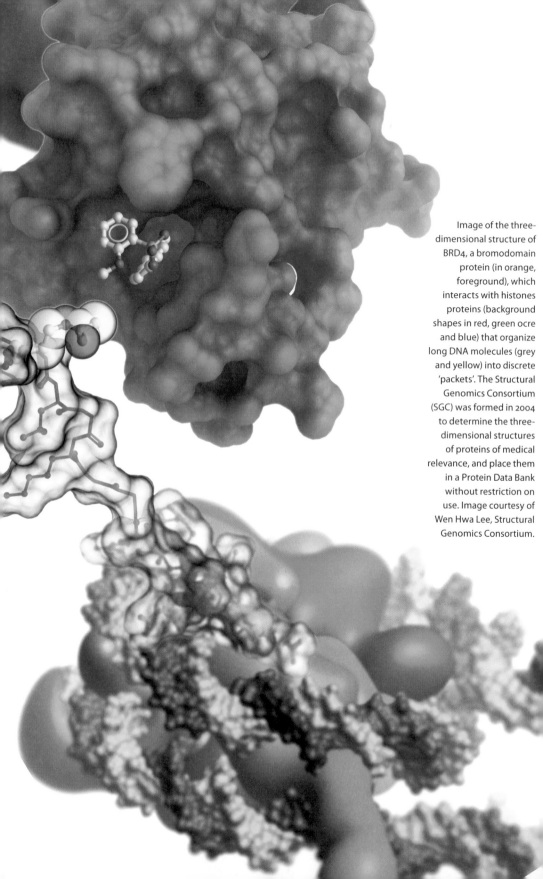

Image of the three-dimensional structure of BRD4, a bromodomain protein (in orange, foreground), which interacts with histones proteins (background shapes in red, green ocre and blue) that organize long DNA molecules (grey and yellow) into discrete 'packets'. The Structural Genomics Consortium (SGC) was formed in 2004 to determine the three-dimensional structures of proteins of medical relevance, and place them in a Protein Data Bank without restriction on use. Image courtesy of Wen Hwa Lee, Structural Genomics Consortium.

The future of drug discovery

Structural Genomics Consortium (SGC)

The discovery of antibiotics has transformed perceptions of medicine's possibilities. But, with the possible exceptions of polio, smallpox and guinea worm, no human disease has been eradicated. It can take ten to fifteen years to find a medicine that works and is safe, at a typical cost of over £1 billion. With pharmaceuticals companies experiencing rapidly declining profits and leaving their home markets, discovering new drugs to treat human disease is becoming an increasingly intractable problem.

Chas Bountra, chief scientist at the Structural Genomics Consortium at the University of Oxford, is at the forefront of contemporary attempts to discover the drugs of the future. He is under no illusion about how difficult the task at hand is. 'It will need a change in the eco-system of the industry. Our job is to solve the structures of human proteins of medical relevance and place them into the public domain without restriction. I want a free-for-all that supports the discovery of new medicines. But the problem of drug discovery is that it is just so incredibly difficult, we don't understand biology well enough.'[73] Indeed, the causes of many diseases still elude us, as do their prevention and cure. Bountra had a long history of working in the pharmaceuticals industry before entering the academic world, and now aims to build on Oxford's celebrated reputation in structural biology. What is currently holding back drug discovery in the biomedical world is secrecy, competition and the strictures of intellectual property. His goal is to dissolve the demarcation lines between industry and academia, and to train the next generation of scientists to work productively on behalf of society and the economy. Barriers need to be broken down and new targets for drug discovery made.

In the human body there are around 22,000 proteins, each of which could potentially be a target for drug discovery, yet only a handful have been studied by scientists. Furthermore, there are hundreds of diseases and hundreds more sub-diseases of which we have only rudimentary knowledge. Academia is not necessarily innovative: researchers cluster around the same proteins, financed by funding agencies that favour established yet unproductive fields rather than innovative but unproven projects. In a bid to avoid what Bountra illuminatingly describes as 'everyone working under the lamp-post', his chosen pathway is basic science – translational patient-orientated research, working with clinicians in hospitals.[74] In this way, understanding protein behaviour has practical application outside the laboratory, and can be used to better appreciate the factors that lead to many common diseases, such as cancer, diabetes, obesity and Alzheimer's. Increasingly, the work being carried out at the SGC is seen as 'game changing' and may well produce a revolution in drug discovery.[75] Oxford science stands at the threshold of a new era, when it may be possible to find a cure for the major diseases of Western society. For Bountra, the challenge is truly formidable: 'discovering a drug for Alzheimer's disease … will be tougher than getting a man onto the moon'.[76]

The state-of-the-art laboratory of the Structural Genomics Consortium, University of Oxford, 2013. Image courtesy of Peter Canning, Structural Genomics Consortium.

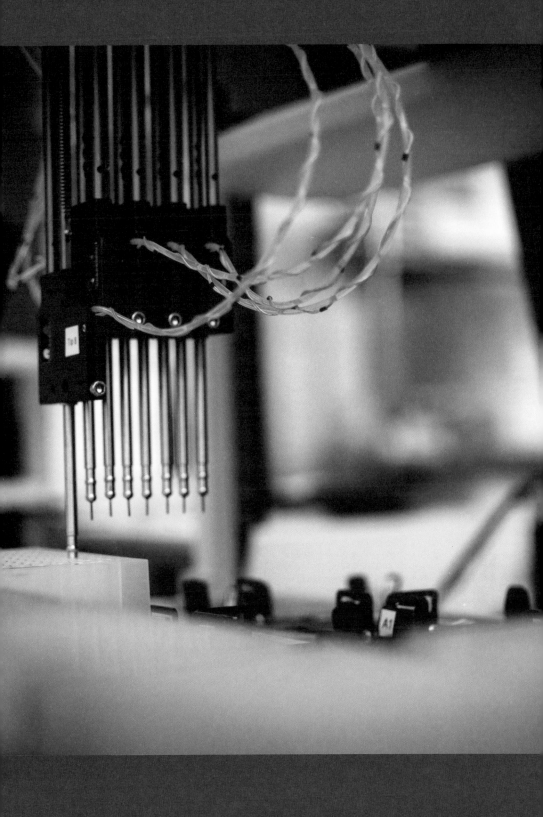

notes

1   C. Webster, *The Great Instauration: Science, Medicine and Reform 1626-1660*, Macmillan, London, 1975.

2   C. Snow, Rede Lecture, 7 May 1959.

3   P. Medawar, *The Art of the Soluble: Creativity and Originality in Science*, Methuen, London, 1967.

4   D. Weatherall, '*The Role of Nature and Nurture in Common Diseases: Garrod's Legacy*', The Harveian Oration, 1992, Royal College of Physicians.

5   *Dictionary of National Biography*, vol. 1, Smith, Elder & Co., London, 1908, p. 847.

6   R. Bacon, *Opera quaedam hactenus inedita*, ed. J. Brewer, Cambridge University Press, Cambridge, 2012, pp. 393–511.

7   *Dictionary of National Biography*, p. 847.

8   Alchemy, within the scheme of knowledge of the period 1200–1650, was in harmony with classical theories of substance, the parallel between the seven known metals and the seven planets, and Aristotelian ideas of growth and becoming. Alchemists sought to accelerate the natural processes that were happening naturally in the earth (A. Chapman, personal communication). Isaac Newton (1642–1727) dedicated much of his time to alchemy.

9   J.H. Bridges (ed.), *The 'Opus Majus' of Roger Bacon*, Oxford, 1897, vol. 1, part II, pp. 56–7.

10 S. Johnson, *Lives of the English Poets*, Clarendon Press, Oxford, 1905, vol. 2, p. 236.

11 C. Severn and H. Colburn (eds), *Diary of the Rev. John Ward, A.M. (1648–1679)*, London, 1839, p. 242.

12 M. Greenwood, 'Sydenham as an epidemiologist', in *Proceedings of the Royal Society of Medicine*, vol. 12, 1919, pp. 55–76

13 A. Chapman, personal communication.

14 C. Webster, *The Great Instauration: Science, Medicine and Reform 1626–1660*, Macmillan, London, 1975, p. 170.

15 A. Chapman, *England's Leonardo: Robert Hooke and the Seventeenth-Century Scientific Revolution*, Institute of Physics Publishing, Bristol, 2005, p. 107.

16 Ibid., p. 51.

17 J. Aubrey, *Brief Lives*, ed. O. Dick, Secker & Warburg, London, 1949, p. 165.

18 T. Wright, *Circulation: William Harvey's Revolutionary Idea*, Chatto & Windus, London, 2012, p. 187.

19 Ibid., p. xi.

20 Ibid., p. 107.

21 J. Simmons, *Doctors and Discoveries: Lives that Created Today's Medicine from Hippocrates to the Present*, Houghton Mifflin, Boston MA, 2002, p. 45.

22 W. Harvey, *The Circulation of the blood and Other Writings*, ed. K. Franklin, Blackwell Scientific, Oxford, 1958, p. 59.

23 A. Larner, 'A Portrait of Richard Lower', *Endeavour*, New Series, vol. 11, no. 4, 1987, pp. 205-8.

24 K. Dewhurst (ed.), *Oxford Medicine: Essays on the Evolution of the Oxford Clinical School to Commemorate the Bicentenary of the Radcliffe Infirmary 1770–1970*, Sandford Publications, Oxford, 1970.

25 N. Williams, *A Pindariqve elegy on the most famous and learned phystian Dr. Willis*, Oxford, 1675, p. 2.

26 He took the name from the village in Oxfordshire where he settled.

27 R. Gunderman, *We Make a Life by What We Give*, Indiana University Press, Bloomington, 2008, p. 56.

28 P. Andrews and E. Brunner, *The Life of Lord Nuffield: A Study in Enterprise and Benevolence*, Blackwell, Oxford, 1953, p. 292.

29 G. Fraenkel, *Hugh Cairns: First Nuffield Professor of Surgery*, Oxford University Press, Oxford, 1991, pp. 101–2.

30 A maximum of three people can share a Nobel Prize.

31 J. Gowans, personal communication.

32 H. Harris, *Oxford Magazine* 158, Second Week Michaelmas Term, 1998, pp. 1–5.

33 M. Heatley, personal communication.

34 *The Mould, The Myth and The Microbe*, BBC Horizon, aired 27 January 1986.

35 H. Harris, 'Howard Florey and the Development of Penicillin', *Notes and Records of the Royal Society of London*, vol. 53, no. 2, 1999, p. 249.

36 G. Ferry, *Dorothy Hodgkin: A Life*, Granta, London, 1999, p. 8

37 Ibid., p. 402.

38 A. Rich, 'Inflammation in Resistance to Infection', *Archives of Pathology*, 22, 1936, p. 228.

39 J. Gowans, personal communication.

40 The Nobel Prize in Physiology or Medicine in 1960 was awarded jointly to Sir Frank Macfarlane Burnet and Peter Brian Medawar 'for the discovery of acquired immunological tolerance'.

41 I. Weissman, 'Lymphocytes, Jim Gowans and *in vivo veritas*', *Nature Immunology*, vol. 11, no. 12, 2010, p. 1073.

42 Karolinska Institute Press Release, 2012, www.nobelprize.org/nobel_prizes/medicine/laureates/2012/press.html accessed 13 June 2013

43 C. Graham, personal communication.

44 J. Gurdon, 'The Developmental Capacity of Nuclei Taken from Intestinal Epithelium Cells of Feeding Tadpoles', *Journal of Embryology and Experimental Morphology*, vol. 10, no. 4, 1962, pp. 622–640.

45 C. Graham, personal communication.

46 A. McMichael, personal communication.

47 C. Graham, personal communication.

48 C. Keating, *Smoking Kills: The Revolutionary Life of Richard Doll*, Signal Books, Oxford, 2009, p. 274.

49 J. O'Connor, personal communication.

50 Ibid.

51 Ibid.

52 P. Williams, personal communication

53 *The Lancet*, 366, 2005, pp. 717–25.

54 *The Lancet*, 376, 2010, pp. 1647–57.

55 *Times Higher Education World University Rankings*, 2011–2012: www.timeshighereducation.co.uk/world-university-rankings/2011-12/subject-ranking/subject/clinical-pre-clinical-health, accessed 1 December 2012.

56 A. Garrod, *Inborn Errors of Metabolism*, Hodder & Stoughton, London, 1909, pp. 5–20.

57 R. Briggs, A. Douglas, R. Macfarlane, J. Gacie, W. Pitney, C. Merskey and J. O'Brien, 'Christmas Disease: A Condition Previously Mistaken for Haemophilia', *British Medical Journal*, vol. 2, no. 4799, 1952, pp. 1378-82.

58 G. Brownlee, personal communication.

59 D. Anson, D. Austen and G. Brownlee, 'Expression of active human clotting factor XI from recombinant DNA Clones in Mammalian Cells', *Nature*, vol. 315, no. 6021, 1985, pp. 683–5.

60 Statement by Barbara Young, chief executive of Diabetes UK, www.diabetes.org.uk/ About_us/News_Landing_Page/Number-of-people-diagnosed-with-diabetes-reaches- three-million, accessed 13 June 2013.

61 A. Hill, personal communication.

62 Ibid.

63 S. Yusuf, R. Collins and R. Peto, 'Why Do We Need Some Large, Simple Randomized Trials?', *Statistics in Medicine*, vol. 3, no. 4, 1984, pp. 409–20.

64 'ISIS-2 (Second International Study of Infarct Survival) Collaborative Group Randomised Trial Of Intravenous Streptokinase, Oral Aspirin, Both, or Neither among 17, 187 Cases of Suspected Acute Myocardial Infarction', *The Lancet*, vol. 332, no. 8607, 1988, pp. 349–60.

65 P. Slight, 'Trials and tribulations: the ISIS experience', *Australian and New Zealand Journal of Medicine*, 22, 1992, pp. 583–5.

66 R. Collins, personal communication,

67 E. Addley, 'Inventor's 2020 Vision: To Help 1bn of the World's Poorest See Better', *Guardian*, 22 December 2008.

68 J. Silver, personal communication.

69 A. Bron, personal communication.

70 A.B. Hill, *Controlled Trials: A Symposium*, Blackwell Scientific, Oxford, 1960, p. 4.

71 I. Chalmers, personal communication.

72 Ibid.

73 C. Bountra, personal communication.

74 Ibid.

75 K. Davies, personal communication.

76 C. Bountra, personal communication.